W9-BUI-077

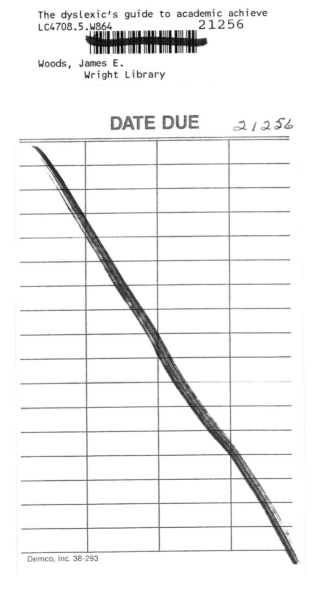

DATE DUE   21256

Demco, Inc. 38-293

THE DYSLEXIC'S GUIDE TO ACADEMIC ACHIEVEMENT

BY

JAMES E. WOODS

ISBN # 1-888321-01-6

CONTENTS

ACKNOWLEDGEMENTS

Throughout the years, the author has experienced many situations which have required the formulation and implementation of strategies in order to overcome opposition. This book is based upon these strategies and the reasoning processes which were necessary to prevail during trying times.

The author wishes to dedicate this book to the teachers and administrators within the American education system who opposed his efforts to receive an education from which to utilize his abilities.

To the Siberian officials from whom the author has received practical experience in the art of bureaucracy manipulation.

Finally, to the few high school and college teachers and administrators who believed in the author's ability to learn and excel in academic studies.

This book is testimony to the fact that strength may be derived from opposition as well as cooperation.

ABOUT THE AUTHOR

JAMES E. WOODS graduated from The University of Texas at Austin on May 20, 1989 with a grade-point-average of 3.23 and a bachelors degree in Organizational Communication. This event was significant, not as a result of his successful completion of academic course work, but rather because he was the first dyslexic student at The University of Texas at Austin to receive all necessary accommodations for dyslexia. It was also significant because he had succeeded in spite of an academic history which was not uncommon for dyslexic students during his time.

He was required to attend special schools from the third to ninth grades which allegedly treated dyslexia. These schools provided virtually no academic challenges and approached dyslexia as though it were a mental handicap.

He reentered the public school system in 1981 and attended the Business and Management Center High School in Dallas. Unaware of his rights to receive accommodations in course work, he devised strategies which he used to overcome academic obstacles in order to graduate fourteenth out of a senior class of 212 in 1984.

James Woods has achieved academic success as a result of his ability to maneuver within the education system. The same ability allowed him to operate a salvage business from the age of eight and to survive for three years in the Irkutsk region of Siberia in spite of overwhelming opposition.

He currently organizes the international marketing of self-help books from his home in Dallas, Texas.

INTRODUCTION

Throughout the course of history, periods of innovation have brought significant improvements to the human condition. These improvements have come as a result of the efforts of individuals who struggled to overcome opposition from institutions which opposed change in order to maintain control during these times. A pattern has arisen over the centuries in which innovative individuals have been persecuted by institutions for their beliefs and efforts to implement change.

Until the late nineteenth century, the term "dyslexia" did not exist and the condition, which contemporary institutions would have us believe to be a disability, was explained as absent-mindedness or eccentricity on the part of dyslexics who had learned to utilize their natural abilities. Dyslexics who failed to realize their true potentials were relegated by society to perform menial tasks without any prospect to develop or benefit from their natural abilities.

Extensive research has been conducted into the causes and possible treatments for dyslexia during this century with contradictory results. The condition, which researchers had initially hoped to isolate and "cure", has proven to be as complicated as the human mind itself. The general understanding of the origins of dyslexia and its effects on the individual are currently limited as a result of research which has provided no conclusive answers.

The Dyslexic's Guide To Academic Achievement relates to history because history is in the making. Although the human condition has advanced further during this century than at any previous time, there still exists opposition to innovation from within institutions which wish to maintain influence. Just as philosophers and inventors have been persecuted for their beliefs throughout history, so too may the dyslexic experience opposition in modern society for his attempts to reform and innovate.

This book has been written to help the dyslexic understand himself and his environment. The techniques which are discussed within will instruct the dyslexic to develop and utilize his natural abilities in order to live a more productive and fulfilling life. It provides a realistic analysis of dyslexia and the environment in which the dyslexic must function in order to succeed. The mission of this book is to eliminate misconceptions which the dyslexic may have acquired regarding his capabilities and to replace them with a mere glimpse into the potential which he holds within his own mind.

This book is not an instructions manual for the dyslexic to use in order to conform to established school policy or to adapt to fit someone else's image of the ideal student. To the contrary, the information contained within this book will explain how the dyslexic student may prompt the school to adapt its policies to suit his needs. It has been written solely for the benefit of the dyslexic student and, while it is not intended to criticize those whose actions have historically been detrimental to dyslexic students, at the same time, it does not offer praise where such expressions are unwarranted.

The information contained within this book is provided in an academic context because the dyslexic must prevail in educational institutions in order to facilitate his efforts to succeed in life. The procedures and recommendations which are provided will easily apply to institutions other than high school and college. As a result, this book should benefit the dyslexic throughout his school years and beyond.

The Dyslexic's Guide To Academic Achievement is a guide to the future; a future in which the dyslexic may use his abilities to overcome opposition in life and strive to achieve goals efficiently and effectively.

Chapter One
THE MEANING OF DYSLEXIA

What is dyslexia if not a disability? There are many schools of thought on this subject which offer conflicting views. To date, an extensive volume of material has been written about dyslexia in order to explain its origins and how it pertains to learning. The word "dyslexia", which is literally defined as "poor or inadequate verbal language", is a good illustration of the extent to which ambiguity has been applied to this particular condition. To define dyslexia in such a fashion is roughly equivalent to defining "The Mona Lisa" as "paint on canvas".

DYSLEXIC THOUGHT PROCESSES

Dyslexia is the result of a superior mind which attempts, and fails, to learn in accordance with methods of teaching which are not conducive to the dyslexic's normal thought processes. These teaching methods are relied upon by modern educational systems and serve to stifle, and in some cases prevent, the dyslexic from learning subjects which are well within his ability to comprehend if taught properly. When a dyslexic student is expected to learn a subject which is taught in a manner that conflicts with his thought processes, problems occur naturally as a result of his attempts to learn the information using dyslexic thought processes. These processes cause him to derive a different, and often incomprehensible, meaning than that which is intended. This inability to correctly comprehend information which is readily understood by non-dyslexics causes many problems for the dyslexic student, both academic and personal.

At the heart of the problem (or the benefit, depending on the reader's point of view) is the fact that dyslexics think differently from non-dyslexics. These dyslexic thought processes are superior to those of non-dyslexics because they provide the dyslexic with considerable advantages if he learns how to utilize them.

DYSLEXIC THOUGHT PROCESSES AS AN OBSTACLE TO READING AND WRITING

The dyslexic mind uses pictorial thought processes while the non-dyslexic mind thinks verbally in a linear fashion. What this means when a dyslexic learns to read is that his mind stores pictures to correspond with each word he learns. For each new word, an additional picture is stored for future reference. The non-dyslexic mind uses a verbal/linear thought process which causes it to mentally visualize the words in a sentence and sound each letter of every word to memorize the information the sentence contains.

The dyslexic encounters problems when reading and writing because many words do not have corresponding pictures and the dyslexic mind is unable to make sense of them. When this happens, the dyslexic experiences a state of confusion which his mind attempts to alleviate through the use of pictorial thought. If the word is incorrectly learned, the dyslexic will misunderstand the word every time he reads it in a sentence.

Lets assume that a dyslexic student attempts to learn the word "not" in class. Although a definition may be found in any dictionary, the dyslexic mind will be unable to comprehend this word because it cannot find a corresponding picture to associate with it. The inability to define the word "not" will cause the dyslexic student to experience confusion as well as frustration. In response, the dyslexic mind will search for a way to apply a picture to the word "not" in order to alleviate the confusion and frustration which the dyslexic student experiences.

Now lets assume that the class ends and the dyslexic student goes to the library to look up the word "not" in the dictionary. He finds the definition, but still cannot understand the word because the dictionary provides him with no means to express the word pictorially. Disgusted, he leaves the library and tries to concentrate on some other subject.

While leaving the library, the dyslexic student sees a sign which reads "Smoking not permitted beyond this point". Although he may only glance at this sign, his mind focuses on the word "not" and subconsciously attempts to provide a pictorial meaning. The sign provides clues to the dyslexic mind through other definable words which are present in the sentence. The word "smoking" may be defined pictorially because the dyslexic student has seen smoke in many forms during his life. The phrase "beyond this point" may also be visualized because the dyslexic student can see the point where the sign hangs and he knows from past experience the meaning of the word "beyond" because he can visualize physically passing a definite point at a time when the word was used. The word "permitted" may also be defined pictorially due to its use in class by a teacher whose image may be visualized in order to give the word meaning.

Through the process of elimination, the dyslexic mind defines all words in the sign with the exception of the word "not". The only task remaining is to examine the environment for stimuli which will provide a definition for the word. While leaving the building, the dyslexic student sees a man sitting on a bench smoking a cigarette. The dyslexic mind examines this picture in an attempt to define the illusive word. The man sits beyond the building's point of exit. His cigarette emits smoke and people pass him on the sidewalk without complaint. At this point, the dyslexic mind incorrectly defines the word "not" pictorially as "a man who sits on a bench". The sign now makes sense to the dyslexic mind: Smoking (the cigarette emits smoke from) not (a man who sits on a bench) permitted (while no one attempts to stop him) beyond this point (further than the exit of the building).

From this point forward, the dyslexic student will visualize a man who sits on a bench every time he reads the word "not". The result of the inconsistency which exists between the meaning of the word and the picture that the dyslexic mind has applied to it will cause the dyslexic student to experience great confusion and frustration in the future. To further complicate the matter, the dyslexic mind has subconsciously performed the process of defining the word, so the dyslexic student cannot explain why he visualizes a man sitting on a bench every time he reads the word "not".

The dyslexic mind will define every word which it cannot pictorially visualize in the same manner as I have just described. The resulting condition will be one in which the dyslexic student cannot understand the meaning of a sentence due to the fact that he is bombarded by inconsistent images which result from words which his mind has incorrectly defined pictorially. At this point, the dyslexic mind will once again perform a process of elimination to determine which words it has incorrectly defined.

When reading a sentence, the dyslexic mind will isolate all words which it has not been able to pictorially visualize and attempt once again to define them. Aware that these words may be incorrectly defined by examining their relation to other words in a sentence, the dyslexic mind will visualize each word as though it were an object from all points of view in an attempt to obtain the illusive meaning.

One of two results will come from this process. First, the dyslexic student will transpose letters in the words due to his mind's attempt to visualize them in an order other than the one in which they appear. This transposition will prevent the dyslexic student from writing the words correctly due to the fact that their letters are organized one dimensionally while he has visualized them three dimensionally in an attempt to define the words. Second, the dyslexic student may incorrectly write the words if his mind succeeds in finding an alternate meaning by reorganizing their letters. In this case, when the dyslexic encounters the word "was", which has no pictorial definition, he will instinctively read and write the word "saw", which his mind will define pictorially as "a tool used for cutting".

Regardless of which process the dyslexic mind performs, the result will be the same, and the dyslexic student will be unable to define the words in question. From this point, the dyslexic mind may simply ignore these words when they are encountered during reading. As a result, when the dyslexic student must answer a question on an exam which asks him to identify something which does not belong, he will subconsciously eliminate the word "not" from the question and experience confusion because all but one of the options given as potential answers will correctly answer the question as he understands it.

DYSLEXIA AND THE OBSTACLE OF LANGUAGE INCONSISTENCY

In addition to reading problems which result from the dyslexic's inability to define words for which no pictorial equivalent exists, he will also experience difficulty when reading words that do not conform to the rules of language as taught in school. Modern English is greatly influenced by words which have been incorporated from other languages that have different rules of spelling and pronunciation. At the same time, correct spelling of all English words is emphasized in school when students learn to read and write. The dyslexic student faces an insurmountable paradox when learning to read the English language because he is given a set of spelling rules to follow in order to learn a language which does not conform to these rules. For example, the word "vacuum" contains "uu" which makes the sound "oo", yet it would be incorrect for the dyslexic student to spell the word "cartoon" using "uu". He must remember that only in the word "vacuum" does the "uu" exist and that it makes the sound "oo". He must also know that the word "cartoon" is not spelled using other variations of letters, and thus create words such as "cartune" or "cartuen".

The problem of spelling for dyslexic students is further complicated by the fact that the English language contains many words which are similar or identical in sound and spelling, yet have different meanings. Consider the following sentence: "You are so close to the clothes hamper, so close the door". This sentence will create numerous difficulties for the dyslexic student due to the fact that the words "close" and "close" are identical in spelling, yet different in sound due to the fact that they reflect a variation on the rules of the English language. Also, the word "so" is used twice in the sentence to convey different messages, even though the spelling and the pronunciation of the word are identical for both usages. The sentence is also confounding for the dyslexic student because the word "clothes" is identical in sound to the verb "close" which the dyslexic would instinctively spell as "cloze" in accordance with the spelling rules he has learned regarding the English language. The only way in which the dyslexic student may learn to spell words which conflict with the rules of the English language is to memorize them. This task often proves to be impossible, given the vast number of words which conflict with the rules of the English language, and therefore, many dyslexics never master the ability to spell.

DYSLEXIA AND STRESS REDUCTION

Without an accurate comprehension of the English language, the dyslexic student will frequently experience stress when reading. This stress is directly proportionate to the complexity of the written material which must be read. If the subject of the written material may be expressed pictorially, the dyslexic student will experience a higher level of comprehension than if the material is expressed abstractly. For this reason, a history class might be more enjoyable for the dyslexic student than a calculus class which teaches subject matter based on abstract principles.

The dyslexic student's subconscious mind contains a mechanism to reduce stress which results from the reading of perplexing written material. When the dyslexic student reads such material, his subconscious mind will focus on a familiar geographical location. This location may originate from the dyslexic student's distant memory and may hold no special appeal, however, it exists to prevent over-concentration on the written material in order to improve his comprehension. The benefits of this subconscious image are two-fold. First, the image reduces stress by providing the dyslexic student a reference to familiar stimuli from the past. Second, the image provides a pictorial reference from which the material may be studied at a later date. If the dyslexic student studies perplexing written material for which his subconscious mind provides a familiar image, the material may be remembered simply by focusing on the various aspects of this image.

DYSLEXIA AND HANDWRITING

Handwriting is considered to be a major problem for dyslexics because it is often illegible to those who must read it. Professors frequently complain that a dyslexic student's handwriting is "messy" or "sloppy", and as a result, they are unable to adequately assess his knowledge of the course material. Professors are then amazed when the dyslexic student reads his own handwriting without difficulty after they have been confounded to find a meaning.

Poor handwriting is not a disadvantage of dyslexia, but rather a manner in which the dyslexic mind deals with a language in which inconsistencies abound. The dyslexic student realizes that he must correctly spell words in order to convey his understanding of the English language, however at the same time, his subconscious mind searches for ways in which he may avoid the rote memorization of every English word which conflicts with the rules he has been taught. The solution to this problem comes early in the education process when the dyslexic student is taught to write cursive, or longhand, English. Regardless of the number of letters, cursive handwriting requires that they all be connected when writing a word. Cursive handwriting allows the dyslexic to subconsciously circumvent the process of sorting words which conform to the rules of the English language and those which do not.

Much to the chagrin of their professors, dyslexic students subconsciously write the English language pictorially through cursive handwriting in order to avoid the problems associated with spelling. A printed word creates problems for the dyslexic student because it is comprised of separate components, or letters, which must be organized in a specific order to provide the correct spelling. The same word spelled cursively consists of only one component which is the sum of all letters connected in a given order. However, variations in the shapes of cursive letters are more limited than their printed counterparts. Therefore, it is more difficult to determine if a cursive word has been misspelled than one which has been printed. (see figure 1.1)

The dyslexic mind will identify a word which has been written in cursive and view it as a shape rather than a series of connected letters. Every time the dyslexic student writes a word in cursive, his mind will ignore the different letters and simply draw the shape which corresponds to the word in question. In this way, the dyslexic mind succeeds in eliminating the need to organize letters in a given order by pictorially representing the word. The dyslexic will instinctively understand the subtle differences between words which have been represented pictorially, while another reader may believe the words to be identical. (see figure 1.2)

THE THREE CATEGORIES OF CURSIVE LETTERS

Category #1
Tall Letters (B,D,H,K,L)

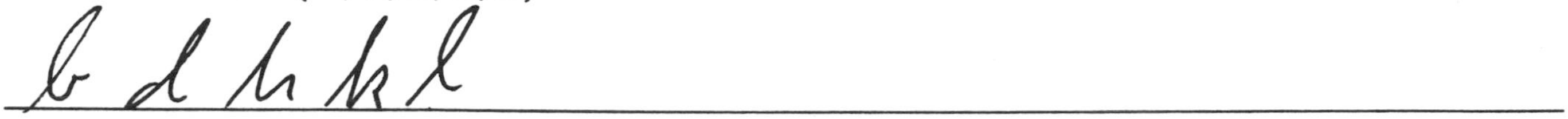

_b d h k l_

Category #2
Short Letters (A,C,E,I,M,N,O,R,S,T,U,V,W,X)

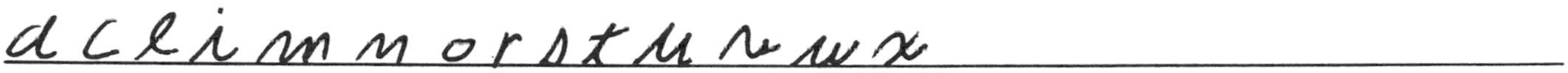

_a c e i m n o r s t u v w x_

Category #3
Low Letters (F,G,J,P,Q,Y,Z,)

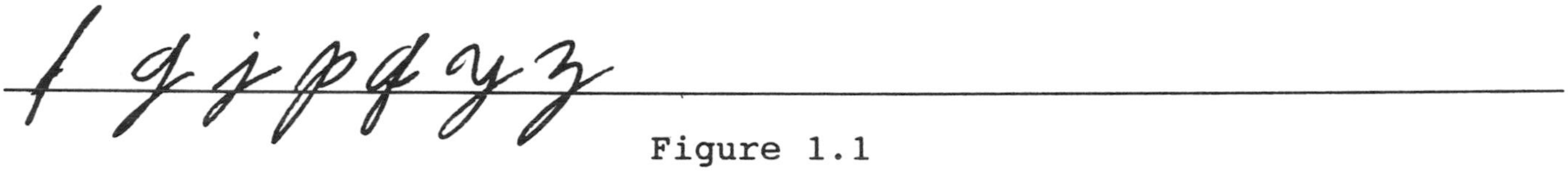

_f g j p q y z_

Figure 1.1

WORDS REPRESENTED PICTORIALLY THROUGH CURSIVE WRITING

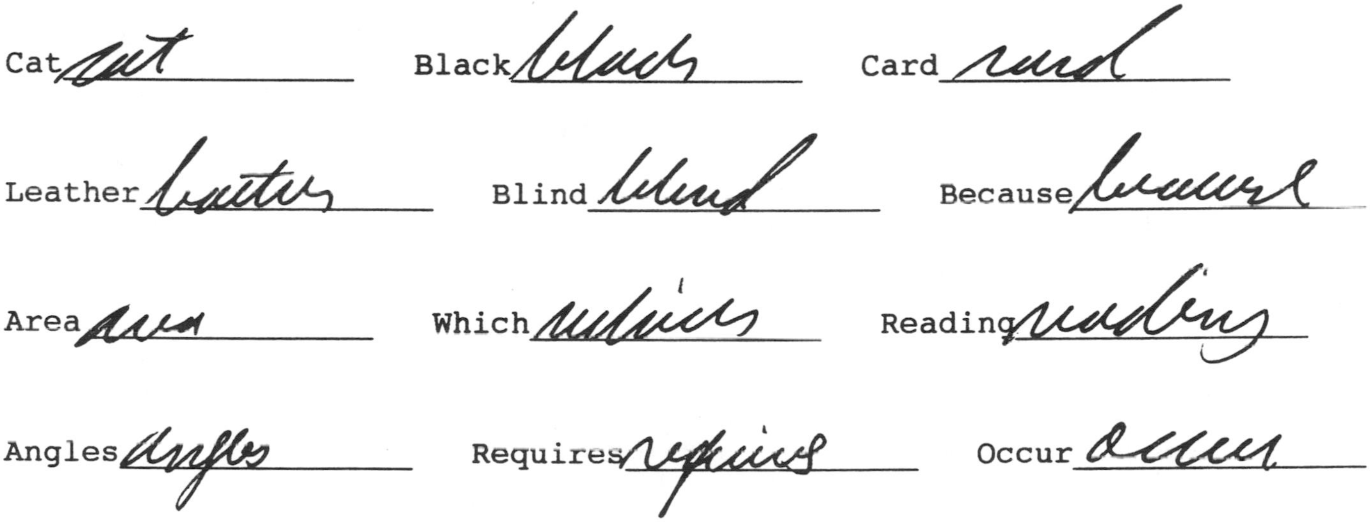

Cat _cat_   Black _black_   Card _card_

Leather _leather_   Blind _blind_   Because _because_

Area _area_   Which _which_   Reading _reading_

Angles _angles_   Requires _requires_   Occur _occur_

* Due to similarities in the cursive letters used by dyslexics, it is
often difficult for the reader to distinguish one word from another.
Analyze the cursive representations above to determine how many
different words could be misinterpreted from each example.

FIGURE 1.2

The process of pictorially representing cursive handwriting may be viewed as the dyslexic mind's response to a language which does not conform to its own rules. In this case, the problem of comprehension is diverted away from the dyslexic student, who perfectly understands his pictorial representations of words, to the professor, who is unable to distinguish one word from another. For the professor, having to read an assignment which has been written by a dyslexic whose mind has converted cursive handwriting into pictorial representation may be equivalent to his having to read an assignment which has been written in Egyptian hieroglyphics.

PICTORIAL THOUGHT AND CREATIVITY

For the dyslexic, comprehension is rarely a problem, but rather the problem is the system which he must follow in order to achieve comprehension. The dyslexic mind is extremely creative and succeeds in finding creative means by which to overcome obstacles, even though the dyslexic may not be consciously aware that these problem-solving processes occur. The dyslexic mind functions many times faster than the non-dyslexic mind which relies on verbal/linear thought processes and allows the dyslexic to pictorially represent thoughts for the purpose of understanding his environment.

Let us say, for example, that a one-minute television excerpt conveys the image of two men who walk down a street, are passed by two cars, and then fall to the ground to avoid being hit by bullets which ricochet off of a sign post. Pictorial thinking allows the dyslexic to view this excerpt in slow motion, regular speed, or rapidly at will. It also allows him to change the sequence of events, add events, or eliminate events to derive a completely different outcome. In the time it would take a person to comprehend the events of the original one minute in a verbal/linear fashion, the dyslexic could not only have comprehended the excerpt, but also altered it and mentally conceived of several subsequent minutes of action which might have followed.

Pictorial thought is perhaps the greatest ability which a dyslexic possesses because it allows him to experience life from more than one dimension. When the dyslexic visualized the two men walking down the street in the previous example, he imagined the scene so completely that it seemed as though he was actually there. He recalled images of scenes which he had encountered in situations similar to the one which he imagined and organized the different components of these past experiences to create a new scene. Although the dyslexic has the ability to distinguish reality from fantasy, the fact remains that he may experience thought as though it were reality. This dyslexic ability has led to great advancements in science which have been achieved by dyslexics who used their pictorial thought processes to create new technologies by combining known components. It has also led to the creation of numerous masterpieces by dyslexics who pictorially imagined the works of art beforehand.

DYSLEXIA VERSUS TRADITIONAL METHODS OF TEACHING

Dyslexia presents three serious problems with respect to traditional forms of teaching. First, the dyslexic mind is selective and will focus attention only on stimuli which it considers to be of most interest. Second, the dyslexic learns subconsciously and is unable to comprehend methods of teaching which lead to a conclusion through rote procedures. Third, the dyslexic mind does not perceive time evenly and is unable to accurately accomplish tasks which are based on a chronological order which is used by non-dyslexics who experience verbal/linear thought processes.

The dyslexic student should be highly valued by educational institutions because his mind automatically focuses attention on the most interesting stimuli it encounters. This ability allows the dyslexic to filter distractions and focus his energy on tasks which are of greatest importance. The problem faced by teachers is that they must structure their lectures in a manner which will be more interesting to the dyslexic student than any other stimuli which reaches his senses during the class period. The teacher must also compete with the imagined stimuli, or alternate reality, which the dyslexic student may automatically create for himself to alleviate boredom which may result from an uninspiring lecture. Many teachers do not possess the communication skills necessary to compete with the dyslexic student's vivid imagination, or even events within the classroom, and never receive the attention of dyslexic students as a result.

Rather than concede the need for improvement in teaching methods, the common practice among educators who fail to inspire dyslexic students is to label them as having Attention Deficit Disorder, or ADD, which places the responsibility for academic failure or underachievement on the dyslexic student. This practice is extremely harmful because such labels create an internal conflict due to the fact that the dyslexic student's subconscious mind is fully aware of its vast capabilities while he may consciously consider himself to be ignorant or stupid as a result of external criticism. Regrettably, a negative self-image caused by such labels will permanently stifle the dyslexic student's ability to succeed in life because his subconscious abilities may only be utilized if he believes that they exist. The irony of this situation is that the dyslexic student who is labeled as having ADD possesses the cognitive ability to master complicated subjects if they are taught in a manner which is conducive to pictorial thinking.

A second problem which dyslexic students face in a traditional educational environment is that their minds work subconsciously to automatically solve problems which non-dyslexic students must solve through standard processes. If nurtured from an early age, a dyslexic may use his subconscious problem-solving abilities to great advantage. However, this development rarely occurs because schools teach subjects to dyslexics in a verbal/linear fashion using steps which non-dyslexics must comprehend in order to reach a conclusion. The dyslexic student, whose mind has the ability to perform these functions subconsciously, is baffled by the procedures required by the teacher to obtain answers to the problems through conscious thought processes. Requiring a dyslexic student to reach a conclusion through rote processes is roughly the same as asking him to explain the muscle contractions which are require in order for him to walk. The process of walking is accomplished through subconscious through in the same manner in which the dyslexic student's mind may automatically solve a problem.

A third problem which dyslexic students face in a traditional educational environment is that they perceive time differently from non-dyslexics due to the fact that they constantly shift their attention from reality to the reality which they create through pictorial thought. Because the dyslexic mind works faster than the non-dyslexic mind, it has the ability to decrease or increase the perceived passage of time to conform to the experiences it creates. If the experiences are interesting to the dyslexic, then the passage of time will seem to increase in order to conform to the level of excitement which the experience produces. If the dyslexic imagines a boring experience, imagined time will appear to elapse slower than normal because his mind is unable to focus on stimuli which appeals to his creative thought processes. If a dyslexic were to image that he was skydiving, for example, he could conceivably experience one minute of imagined time for every three minutes which actually elapse. However, if the dyslexic was to image a clock which hangs on a wall in a silent room where the only movement comes from the second hand, imagined time might pass at the rate of three complete rotations of the second hand for every minute of actual time which elapses.

Time distortion is a characteristic trait of dyslexics and explains why dyslexics often have what educators perceive to be memory problems. For the non-dyslexic, time passes in a constant, linear fashion from which memories are drawn. The dyslexic does not have the ability to gauge the correct passage of time. If a dyslexic experiences excitement during a period of time, he will perceive this time to have been short due to a rapid perception of elapsed time. However, boredom will be perceived as a period of time which is much longer than actual or the dyslexic will create an imagined event during this time which will cause his perception of elapsed time to be either longer or shorter than reality. Regardless, the dyslexic's memory will be a collection of images and events which may have no relation to actual elapsed time. It will also be common for events which have occurred years prior to be remembered as recent events, while recent events may be perceived to have occurred long ago. This is the reason why a dyslexic who has worked at a boring job for three years may believe that he has worked for ten, while at the same time, believe that his college graduation ten years earlier has occurred only three years prior.

When a dyslexic focuses attention on a teacher's lecture, he experiences time at a normal rate of speed. However, if the lecture is not interesting, he will focus his attention on an alternate reality which he perceives through pictorial thought. During the time when he focuses on this alternate reality, time passes at a different rate of speed because the dyslexic mind controls the perceived passing of time which the student experiences. If during a class the dyslexic student becomes bored, he may imagine that he is walking down a street, two cars pass, and bullets ricochet off of a sign post. He may experience several variations of this event or create other events to alleviate the boredom he feels. When he focuses his attention on the lecture once more, he may perceive that ten minutes of actual time have passed, however, actual time has elapsed much faster than he had expected and he finds that the class, which seems to have begun only ten minutes earlier, has come to an end.

TIME DISTORTION AND MATHEMATICS

Time distortion creates great difficulties in mathematics because the procedures which are required to answer mathematical problems are based on a linear passage of time which the dyslexic student has never experienced. The dyslexic student experiences reality, not in a linear fashion, but rather as a constant bombardment of thoughts and images both real and imagined. The concept of mathematical problem-solving presents the dyslexic with an image of reality in which this constant shifting is absent. The dyslexic student is required to focus his attention solely on the steps required to solve the mathematical problem in order to recreate the progression of the linear passing of time which he has never experienced. This attempt results in the dyslexic student concentrating all of his energy on the performance of a task which his brain will not consciously perform until he reaches a point of exhaustion.

A great irony exists with respect to the dyslexic student and mathematical problem-solving because the dyslexic has the ability to subconsciously solve problems without performing the rote steps demanded by the education system. Dyslexic students often find it easier to "guess" the answer to a mathematical question rather than obtain the answer using traditional steps. What these dyslexic students don't realize is that their ability to guess the answer is in reality the dyslexic mind subconsciously solving the problem for them.

If a dyslexic student is required to answer mathematical problems using a multiple choice exam, they often demonstrate this subconscious problem-solving ability by choosing the correct answers from the options given. Unfortunately, teachers who grade these exams usually notice a significant improvement in the dyslexic student's performance in relation to other forms of mathematical testing and accuse him of cheating when he is unable to provide evidence that he has performed the required steps on separate sheets of paper. The teacher's accusation is further reinforced when the dyslexic student fails to explain the process he used to obtain the answers to the exam questions. At this point, the dyslexic student is punished by the teacher for using a unique problem-solving ability which he is not aware exists in place of performing steps which require him to duplicate a passing of time which he has never experienced.

The case of Albert Einstein illustrates the difference between solving mathematical problems subconsciously as opposed to using rote processes. Einstein has come to be regarded as the greatest physicist in history, yet he frequently claimed during his life that he poorly understood mathematics. In the process of solving complex equations, he stated that he viewed himself as a hunter and the solution to his equation was the prey which he pursued. The process of solving the equation required him to overcome the evasive maneuvers of his prey. His prey was captured at the point when he had solved his equation. In this way, Einstein used pictorial thought in order to visualize the equation as an object while his subconscious mind led him to the conclusion which he sought. Ironically, mathematicians throughout the world praise Einstein for his accomplishments while modern education systems stifle the abilities of dyslexic students through the teaching of rote mathematical processes.

DYSLEXIA AS AN INNOVATIVE RESOURCE

The problem of dyslexia results from the inability of a dyslexic mind to pictorially comprehend its environment. The benefit of dyslexia, on the other hand, comes from the ability of the dyslexic mind to pictorially analyze, restructure, and reorganize its environment at such speed that the dyslexic is unaware that this process occurs. The implications of this ability are far-reaching for society if the dyslexic is educated in a manner which will develop, and not stifle, his ability to use pictorial thought processes.

The dyslexic's ability to subconsciously reorganize elements from his environment through pictorial thought processes is perhaps the greatest resource available to mankind. Human existence depends upon the ability of mankind to constantly change in order to adapt to the environment. Imagine a world without medicine in which every disease is allowed to spread and infect the human inhabitants. This world would soon be populated by the dying due to the failure of the human immune systems to combat the invading viruses. Without the ability to pictorially analyze and reorganize elements of the environment, no medicine would ever be produced because mankind would lack the necessary creativity to imagine that a combination of elements could produce a medicine which would kill the viruses after they had entered the body.

During this century, the advancement of technology has increased to the point where mankind is unable to survive without the constant introduction of new technologies. As a result, mankind must rely on the ability of dyslexics to subconsciously create. In spite of having to deal with an education system which has historically been oppressive to dyslexic students' development, notable advancements have been made by many dyslexics which have permanently altered human existence through innovative achievements.

Without the contributions of these notable dyslexics, life as we know it would be much different. Imagine a modern society without telephones. If Alexander Graham bell had never lived, we might never have benefited from the invention of the telephone. The electric light bulb might never have been invented if it had not been for the persistence of Thomas Edison who tested over a thousand different materials to conduct electricity before he found one suitable. Of course, the argument may be made that America could have been destroyed if it had not been for the rapid advancements made by Albert Einstein in the invention of the atomic bomb ahead of his German counterparts during World War II. It is also unlikely that the war in Europe would have ended as quickly without the contributions of General George Patton who possessed an uncanny aptitude for military strategy.

Chapter Two
AN INWARD VIEW

_____

By this time, the reader may have the impression that we are
essentially talking about two identities within one person when we
speak of the dyslexic conscious and subconscious mind. In fact, this
impression is not entirely incorrect because the dyslexic subconscious
mind is much more active than that of a non-dyslexic due to pictorial
thought processes which alleviate much of the conscious thought
processes which the non-dyslexic mind must perform in order to
comprehend its environment. However, this "two in one" impression may
oversimplify a much more complicated psychological relationship due to
the fact that the dyslexic's conscious self-image regulates his
subconscious mind's ability to function. If the dyslexic believes from
an early age that he is "disabled", "slow", or inferior in any way,
his conscious mind will encode this information onto his psyche due to
the fact that he has no contradictory information to counter this
label, and also because he is aware by this time that he has
difficulty to learn subjects which pose no problems to his classmates.

THE INTERNAL CONFLICT OF DYSLEXIA

The dyslexic is his own worst critic in life because he is
subconsciously aware of his vast capabilities, yet he consistently
makes what he considers to be stupid mistakes for which he has no
explanation, and worse, no control. This internal conflict may present
the dyslexic student with a negative self-image in relation to his
peers which will stifle his subconscious mind's ability to function.

The dyslexic student will then be forced into a vicious circle in which his academic performance will continue to deteriorate as his mental capacity for learning becomes increasingly blocked by his inability to perform. The more mistakes he makes, the worse his self-image becomes, and he makes more mistakes as a result.

One of the greatest tasks which the dyslexic student faces is to overcome the tendency to develop a negative self-image. This task is great due to experiences which occur early during grade school years. It is common for dyslexic students to have had conflict with a teacher during grade school who attempted to educate through ridicule. The ridicule theory states that a student will learn when he believes that he will experience embarrassment in the event of failure. This practice is debilitating to the dyslexic student due to his inability to control, or even understand, the subconscious thought processes which place him in a superior position to learn. The subject, for which he makes mistakes during class, is formidable as a result of the teacher's inappropriate method of instruction.

The dyslexic student views the teacher as an authority figure and rarely questions her observations. If the teacher ridicules the dyslexic student in an attempt to teach him a subject, he will adopt a practice of self-ridicule in an effort to overcome his inability to correctly perform required tasks. When this process fails to provide the desired results, the dyslexic student will increase his self-ridicule to the point where his self-image is literally destroyed by negative emotions which cause him to doubt his abilities and his value as a person because he will consciously block any attempts made by his subconscious mind to find alternate methods of performing tasks.

As a cognitive safety mechanism, the subconscious dyslexic mind will provide the dyslexic with a superior ego to combat the effects of self-ridicule which may result from his failure to perform seemingly uncomplicated tasks. This ego allows the dyslexic student to consciously place himself above his peers or the tasks he must perform by deeming them to be insignificant or irrelevant rather than deem himself to be a failure. The dyslexic ego may be developed easily if the dyslexic student has previously accomplished a task quickly in relation to his peers and received praise for it. The conscious mind will accept this information as proof that the dyslexic is not inferior and allow him to maintain a psychological balance between negative influences from his work and positive influences from his accomplishments.

A biographical study of famous dyslexics will reveal that they experienced a continuous battle between these two opposing self-images during their lives. When great accomplishments were achieved, the dyslexic ego was reinforced and the subconscious mind's ability to function was enhanced. However, during the developmental stages which led to these achievements, the dyslexics were besieged by the effects of self-ridicule and doubt regarding the correctness of their actions. In order to combat negative influences, these dyslexics focused their attentions on tasks which they performed to the exclusion of all other influences. This attention to detail caused perceived time to elapse much slower than actual time due to the need to pictorially explore all aspects of the task. Thomas Edison was a classic example of a dyslexic who became engrossed in his thoughts in order to achieve success. He lived in his laboratory and experimented day and night until he found a solution. His wife would bring him meals for nourishment, but she knew that he would be aloof until he had accomplished his goal.

DYSLEXIA AND ACHIEVEMENT

It is necessary for the reader to understand that dyslexia is not limited to reading, writing, and arithmetic. Any function which the dyslexic mind performs may be enhanced subconsciously or stifled consciously. In the case of athletes, subconscious pictorial thought processes allow them to perform physical feats automatically which require the non-dyslexic mind years to master, if at all. Success occurs because pictorial thought allows the dyslexic athlete to visualize ideal movements which are required to achieve athletic goals. Pictorial thought allows a unique harmony to take place between the physical and mental development of the dyslexic athlete. The accomplishments of Jackie Stewart, Bruce Jenner, and Greg Louganis live as testimony to the potential of this unique dyslexic ability.

Dyslexia may also enhance, or inhibit, the ability to relate to other people. The subconscious dyslexic mind is highly analytical and focuses on all stimuli within the environment. When the dyslexic is involved in discourse with other people, his subconscious mind records aspects of the other person's character, actions, and thoughts in order to better understand him. This absorption of information provides the dyslexic with the ability to relate well with people because they have the ability to essentially "see the world through another's eyes".

DYSLEXIA AND INTERPERSONAL RELATIONSHIPS

In the case of interpersonal relationships, dyslexics may experience harmony with their mates due to the ability to anticipate these people's needs and avoid situations which would hold potential conflict. The dyslexic has the ability to use subconscious thought processes to relate to other people and may be selective when choosing a mate because he can easily identify those with whom he would conflict.

As I have already stated, the dyslexic focuses attention on the most interesting stimuli which exists within his environment. If the dyslexic falls in love, he may completely devote himself to his mate in whom he is most interested. This attention may be misinterpreted by observers as infatuation when in fact it is a natural response which occurs as a result of dyslexic thought processes.

There exist three disadvantages of dyslexia with respect to interpersonal relationships.

First, the dyslexic is a unique individual who experiences reality differently than most people. Therefore, the number of potential mates who could understand such a person is limited.

Second, the dyslexic has the ability to create an alternate reality from other people and may, in the absence of a suitable mate, become engrossed in his thoughts and focus attention away from the search for a mate. As always, the people who surround the dyslexic must compete with the reality which he may create for himself. If these people are not interesting to the dyslexic, they may complain that he is aloof, or introverted, when in fact he has simply focused his attention elsewhere.

Third, and most importantly, the dyslexic who finds a suitable mate will experience extreme self-ridicule if this mate fails to share his affections. In order for the dyslexic to fall in love, he must eliminate the psychological defense mechanisms which he has developed to overcome negative self-images caused by failure to perform in accordance with his own expectations. Without these protections, rejection may be a stifling experience which will cause the dyslexic to react in one of four ways:

a) Withdraw into his own thoughts in an attempt to find solace through pictorial thought processes. In this case, the ability to create a separate reality is used in an attempt to escape the pain of rejection long enough for self-ridicule to subside to a level where defense mechanisms may be restored.

b) Combat self-ridicule through actions which alleviate the pain of rejection by reinforcing previous feelings of superiority. In this case, the dyslexic turns his anger outward in an attempt to place himself in a situation which conflicts with his feelings of inadequacy. This situation may be achieved through the manipulation of existing systems within the dyslexic's environment from which he may gain wealth or influence. The need to overcome self-ridicule will become so great that his mind will achieve a heightened state of awareness which will allow him to analyze the relationships between system components in order to influence them to achieve the desired result. Defense mechanisms will be restored when he has proven to himself that he can achieve this desired result and overcome external opposition within his environment. At this point, the existence of opposition which exists internally in the form of self-ridicule will be replaced by self-confidence.

c) Attempt to eliminate self-ridicule through physical exertion. In this case, the dyslexic performs strenuous physical activities in an attempt to eliminate the pain of rejection. A heightened state of awareness results from the determination to achieve athletic goals which continuously require greater levels of physical endurance. This increase in physical activity causes the mind to produce endorphins which counteract feeling of self-ridicule and create the illusion of psychological well-being.
    As the dyslexic becomes engrossed in physical activity, his emotional responses to stimuli which exist within his environment will decrease to the point where he becomes isolated within his own thoughts. The subconscious mind uses pictorial thought to create an alternate reality which consoles the dyslexic until the pain of rejection begins to subside. At this point, physical activity decreases as the dyslexic regains his defense mechanisms and begins to relate to stimuli within his environment.

d) Reinforce self-ridicule through self-destructive behavior. In this case, the dyslexic not only fails to overcome the pain of rejection, but uses the experience of rejection as a catalyst from which to intensify existing feelings of inadequacy. The culmination of negative emotions which have been suppressed over years of failure form a self-image which conflicts with that which the dyslexic held prior to rejection. As a result, the dyslexic views himself as the embodiment of the weakness which he wishes to overcome, thus creating the justification for self-abuse. A cycle appears as the dyslexic continues to punish himself for his failure in love while blocking his subconscious mind's ability to provide a solution to the pain of rejection. The cycle intensifies as the dyslexic's behavior becomes increasingly more severe.

In the early stages, self-destructive behavior may consist of habits such as smoking or drinking. However, as self-ridicule intensifies, these behaviors may evolve into drug abuse or involvement in criminal activities. Eventually, the dyslexic will feel totally isolated from his environment and his subconscious mind will be unable to penetrate the barrier which has been created by negative emotions. A point will eventually be reached where the dyslexic believes that he is no longer affected by events which occur within his environment and he will have no means by which to retreat into his subconscious mind for solace. At this point, self-destructive behavior develops into suicidal tendencies.

Interpersonal relationships pose a greater challenge to the dyslexic than any activity which must be mastered in life because success in love may only be achieved after psychological defense mechanisms have been eliminated. The risks which are present in the event of failure are far more damaging than those associated with academic challenges due to strong emotional attachments which result from interpersonal relationships and vulnerability to the influence of negative emotions.

DYSLEXIA AND TASK COMPLETION

The ability to see the world through another's eyes is beneficial in conflict because the dyslexic may anticipate his opponent's actions and manipulate him through the creation of challenging situations. For this reason, dyslexics often make good arbitrators and lawyers. The dyslexic's ability in any given area will be determined by the needs of his situation. If, as in the case of Thomas Edison, the task is to invent a machine, the dyslexic mind will devote its efforts to creating a physical object. If the task is to defeat an opponent, the dyslexic mind will focus on the opponent's thought patterns to anticipate this person's actions.

The ability to see the world through another's eyes is invaluable in the theater where actors are required to duplicate another person's character. When the dyslexic is familiar with his part, his mind may duplicate the actions and thoughts of another person to the point of convincing the audience that he is actually that person. This ability is not limited to actions and thought, though. A dyslexic may freely impersonate another person's voice or accent perfectly. In this case, the subconscious mind duplicates the sound and pattern of the other person's voice and expresses these changes through speech. Among some of the more famous dyslexic members of the acting profession are Whoopi Goldberg, Cher, and Danny Glover.

Chapter Three
DEVELOPING EFFECTIVE SUCCESS STRATEGIES

If my efforts have been effective to this point, the reader now understands that dyslexia is not a disability but rather an imbalance of abilities caused by the attempts of a mind which thinks pictorially to comprehend stimuli which is presented in a verbal/linear fashion. If the reader is dyslexic, he should have related to much that I have written and now have a better understanding of his present situation and the events which have led to this point. The next question to be answered is "what may be done in order to succeed in college?". The answer to this question is that the reader will use his abilities to overcome the obstacles which are present in the education system.

THE DESTRUCTION OF NEGATIVE SELF-IMAGE

Before the dyslexic student can defeat the opposition which he faces in his environment, he must first overcome the opposition which exists within his own mind. As a dyslexic, he has endured years of inappropriate instruction in order to reach this point in his educational development. As a result, his mind has adopted a natural response of self-criticism to be enacted when he fails to perform in accordance with his own expectations. This self-criticism is a learned response from years of inappropriate instruction by adults who believed that he would learn in order to avoid criticism. Self-criticism must be eliminated in order for the dyslexic student to succeed because it creates a negative self-image which inhibits his subconscious mind from functioning. In this way, the process of self-criticism, which was originally acquired to improve academic performance, will actually curtail performance due to the diminished capacity of the subconscious mind.

In order to overcome a negative self-image caused by self-criticism, the dyslexic student must acquire a correct understanding of his true identity and his place in the environment. Once he understands that he is not disabled, but rather that he possesses cognitive abilities greater than eighty-five percent of the people on this planet, he will begin to understand the extent of his potential.

DYSLEXIA AND THE MODERN EDUCATION SYSTEM

Once the effects of negative self-image have been overcome, the next task will be for the dyslexic student to develop a correct image of himself in relation to the education system. Regardless of his present educational level, he must understand that his inability to perform according to the standards of the education system is a learned condition which he has received from the education system itself. As a dyslexic, his mind has the potential to function hundreds of times faster than the minds of non-dyslexics. The reason why he works slowly, or ineffectually, is because the education system has taught him that performance is gauged on the basis of established procedures which must be followed. These established procedures require predetermined amounts of time to perform. Once accepted, this relationship between procedure and time has caused the dyslexic conscious mind to stifle his natural ability to subconsciously solve problems immediately. The disability of dyslexia lies in the fact that the subconscious dyslexic mind is capable of solving problems while the conscious dyslexic mind is convinced that such an ability does not exist while unsuccessfully attempting to follow the verbal/linear procedures taught by the education system.

The tendency to think in terms of time stifles dyslexic creativity because it creates a mental block in which the dyslexic student believes that creativity is governed by time. If a dyslexic student has always been given exams in which mathematical questions must be answered at the rate of one per minute, he will develop an ingrained belief that one minute will always be required to answer such a question. Albert Einstein has proven that the dyslexic subconscious mind may rapidly solve the most complex mathematical questions if it is allowed to do so without negative influences. While Einstein's subconscious mind solved equations, he viewed the entire process as a hunt in which he was involved. His mind rapidly solved the equations because he viewed the process pictorially as an event which had no relation to mathematics.

The dyslexic student must learn to use his abilities in order to overcome the negative self-image which has developed as a result of his attempts to conform to the education system's processes. For this reason, it will be necessary for the dyslexic student to begin a period of discovery in which he becomes aware of his true potential. The difficulty of this process will depend on the extent of the negative self-image which has resulted from criticism, both internal and external. The period will begin when the dyslexic student develops a positive image of himself in relation to the education system and develops strategies for success.

The main problem which the dyslexic student faces to develop a positive self-image in relation to the education system is that he sees it from an inferior point of view. For the dyslexic, school is a difficult, and even terrifying, experience in which he does not perform satisfactorily and is punished as a result. The thought of school often causes fear which conflicts with his subconscious mind's ability to function due to the fact that negative emotions are associated with the subjects which the dyslexic must learn. In this case, school is actually a de-educational institution because the dyslexic student loses the positive self-image which is required for his subconscious mind to assist him in his course work. After continued failure, the dyslexic student will either work to the point of exhaustion in hopes of succeeding or simply fail and live his life believing that he is a failure due to his inability to succeed in school.

A POSITIVE SELF-IMAGE DEVELOPED FROM A DIFFICULT SITUATION

Due to an unlikely event, I managed to develop a positive image of myself in relation to the education system which allowed me to work successfully in school from an early age. When I attended the third grade, I experienced conflict with a teacher one day who was dissatisfied with my performance in class. Instead of trying to encourage me to understand the material, she ridiculed me and caused me to experience negative feelings about myself. When my father came home from work that night, I told him what had happened. My father, who is also dyslexic, told me that "the teacher was more stupid than she thought I was". He then explained that he had always had problems with school teachers due to his dyslexia. According to my father, there were two types of people in the world: "those who act and those who teach". My father explained to me that, in his opinion, a teacher is a person who has obtained significant knowledge about a given subject, yet lacks the ambition to utilize this knowledge to improve her life. For this reason, according to my father, she passes this knowledge to her students in hopes that they will possess the ambition which she lacks to utilize this knowledge for the good of society.

I considered my father's concept of education to be quite revolutionary, however, I trusted my father's judgment and I began to test his theory. When I returned to school the next day, I observed my teachers to determine if I could find any evidence to support my father's theory of education. I soon began to observe my father's business associates, who were the only other group of adults to whom I had access, to understand their behaviors and characteristics. I spent an entire month watching these two groups of adults in various situations. I observed the teachers in an educational environment daily and often overheard conversations which they had about their private lives during lunch and after class. My father's business associates were also available for me to study when I went to his place of business after school.

After a month, I was surprised to find that my father's theory seemed to be valid. By comparing the two groups of adults, I could tell that distinct differences existed which set them apart from one another. My father's business associates, who worked in the manufacturing industry, seemed to be the more creative group. Their conversations focused mainly on topics related to money and manufacturing. They were independent adults who had the capacity to

19

conceive and build things which I couldn't understand using measurements about which I knew nothing. They all had significant cash reserves available from which to work and they were able to conceive of ways in which this money could be used to obtain profit. When I expressed interest in their topics of conversation and asked questions, they were pleased and went to great lengths to answer my questions in ways that I could understand.

The teachers, on the other hand, held conversations which focused on topics which dealt mainly with current events, television programs, and gossip. I could never tell that anything was ever resolved from their discussions and they were far easier for me to understand than those of the other group. When the topic of the teachers' conversations turned to the subject of money, it usually dealt with the lack of money, rather than the conceptualizing of plans to increase it. There also seemed to be much time devoted to the discussion of interpersonal problems which were absent from the conversations of the other group.

I concluded that my father was correct in his observation of the education system. This conclusion would have far-reaching effects on my educational development because it was at that point that I developed a positive image of myself in relation to the education system. From that point forward, I saw the teacher, not as a figure to be respected or feared, but rather as a person to humored. I came to the conclusion that a teacher's inability to accept my lack of knowledge in a particular subject was not my problem, but rather, an example of her weakness.

From this point, my experiment continued. I had already developed an understanding of "teacher psychology", so the next step was to identify "student psychology". I began to observe my fellow students to determine how they interacted with the teacher both inside and outside of the classroom. I observed that the students usually exhibited characteristics of fantasy in their interaction with one another and that their interaction with the teacher was inhibited when they interjected these characteristics into conversation. The students who the teacher perceived most favorably were those who approached course work from an analytical point of view which they developed by interacting with the teacher to improve their understanding. The teacher's favor for students who learned through interaction seemed logical in the context of my father's theory because this interaction seemed to reinforce the teacher's positive self-image.

When I understood the various characteristics of the groups I studied, I learned that I could induce a response from members of these groups by appealing to their beliefs. I observed that inequality existed in the treatment which students received depending upon the teacher's opinion of each student. Those students who were perceived to be the brightest were given preferential treatment by the teacher while the students who were perceived to be "problem children" would often receive derision in situations for which such treatment was not necessary. I learned that I could induce a desired response from the teacher by responding in a certain way to given situations. I could obtain good results by behaving as one of the bright students, however, I soon learned that I would be perceived even more favorably if I responded to given situations in a manner which reflected teacher psychology. In this way, I managed to develop an empathy with the teacher in which she would perceive me differently from the other children and I would be able to function without the restrictions which were usually present in the teacher-student relationship.

THE POSITIVE SELF-IMAGE AND MANIPULATION

It was at this point that I developed a useful ability as the result of my father's revolutionary theory of education: manipulation. I began to view the school as a system of components which operates based upon written regulations and purposes in theory, while at the same time, is greatly influenced by the personalities and beliefs of its members. I recognized distinct inconsistencies between the public and private views which teachers held for school administrators and vice versa. A certain amount of resentment was often present between these two groups to which I could appeal in order to induce a desired response from members within either group. I began to understand trends in the manner in which different groups interacted with one another and I could predict the outcomes of various situations based upon one group's ability to present its case in accordance with the beliefs which were held by the other group. I learned that I could sit in a classroom and effect a desired change in the course of discussion simply by interjecting comments which either appealed to or conflicted with the beliefs which were held by the teacher and the other students.

I learned that school lessons were based not only on facts but also on the teacher's interpretation of these facts. I found that the teacher would provide a student who she perceived to be knowledgeable with the benefit of the doubt regarding his understanding of the subjects that she taught. For this reason, it was possible for me to be perceived favorably by the teacher and improve my grades simply by presenting course work in a fashion which supported her beliefs. I also learned that, if I remained silent during question periods when I required information, another student would usually ask a question which would provide the information that I needed in order to understand the subject. Without revealing my lack of knowledge, I appeared knowledgeable due to the fact that I asked few questions. As a result, the teacher graded my assignments favorably because she believed that I had an excellent understanding of the subject because I asked few questions during class.

Over the years, I developed an alternate image of the education system as a result of my experimentation. I devised the theory that the education system does not exist solely for the purpose of instilling knowledge into the minds of students, but that it also exists, if not in purpose then definitely in fact, as a precursor to the lives that students will likely lead after graduation. Especially in college, the student encounters a highly bureaucratic system of administration which operates on strict procedures which must be followed in order to succeed. The course work is extensive, and the teachers vary greatly in their approaches to the subjects they teach. Among the teachers and administrators, the student will encounter the traits, both positive and negative, which will be present among administrators in a business environment. The student's ability to deal effectively with these people will determine the likelihood of success after graduation.

During my school years, I held the belief that the education system was a potential source of knowledge, however, I found that I could learn much more through contact with people outside of the educational environment such as my father's business associates. The education which I received in school was limited and governed by time constraints. Course work involved little creativity, but rather, the absorption of facts. My association with adults outside of the educational environment taught me the value of creative thinking which I used to circumvent tedious course work in order to utilize my private time for exercises in experimentation and business management.

My father was an inventor of sorts who owned a company which designed and built parts and machinery from metal. For this reason, my father and his associates were highly creative because their professions required them to conceive and build. When discussing my father's accomplishments one day, he told me that "you can do anything you want in life until someone teaches you how to do it". He went on to explain to me that alternatives usually exist to the procedures which are taught in schools to reach a desired goal. These alternatives, according to my father, are obtainable only if a person attempts to solve a problem without having been influenced by these accepted procedures. If a person approaches a problem from an analytical perspective, his mind subconsciously provides the means to obtain the desired goal only when the conscious mind does not attempt to interject learned procedures.

Again, I received a revolutionary concept from my father which I began to verify in my own life. I quickly found that his conclusion was correct because I could approach tasks for which I had received little instruction and develop methods to reach a conclusion faster than those provided through traditional instruction. I developed the theory that the education system did not exist to promote creativity, but rather, conformity. This theory was supported by observations I had made of the education system's resistance to change and the turmoil which resulted from innovations being introduced due to procedural inflexibility.

THE THREE LEVELS OF CONSCIOUS AWARENESS

As I developed a tendency to experiment in order to determine alternative procedures, I became aware of what I refer to as the three levels of conscious awareness. When I faced a problem which was conveyed in a verbal/linear fashion, I would view it pictorially as being at a point in space which was physically higher than myself. From my position, I was intimidated by the problem and experienced tension as a result of my inability to solve it using pictorial thought processes. I also experienced frequent depression during my teenage years in which I seemed to be underneath a dark cloud which contained all of my problems in life. This first level of conscious awareness was debilitating because it interfered with my subconscious mind's ability to function effectively and I experienced a negative self-image as a result. I particularly experienced this first level of conscious awareness during times when I was required to solve abstract mathematical problems, the processes for which I could not comprehend.

I realized that I viewed mundane tasks as being at a point in space which was physically equal to myself. If drove a car, chose a meal from a menu, or tied my shoes, these tasks would present themselves as being neutral because they were so familiar that I would do them automatically. I found that the majority of my experiences occurred on this neutral level of conscious awareness.

It was only when I began to achieve success through experimentation that I became aware of the third, and most favorable, level of conscious awareness. This third level of conscious awareness placed me at a point where I seemed to be physically above the task which I had to achieve, and from this superior position, my mind worked quickly and efficiently. From this third level of conscious awareness my creativity would literally soar and I could devise methods of problem-solving and obtain inspiration the extent of which I had previously been unaware. My mind would work so quickly that it seemed as though I was automatically acting in areas which previously had required concentration.

My discovery of the three levels of conscious awareness was not original. I later learned that a man name Napoleon Hill had studied the philosophies of many accomplished Americans, such as the Nineteenth-century industrialist Andrew Carnegie, and had come to similar conclusions. In his book, Think And Grow Rich, Mister Hill conceived of a heightened state of mind which could be achieved through the elimination of negative thoughts along with the implementation of instructions into the subconscious mind accompanied by a determination to succeed. When this task had been completed, the subconscious mind, according to Hill, would connect with what he referred to as "Infinite Intelligence" which would cause the subconscious mind to become a receptor for inspiration.

Although I consider Think And Grow Rich to rely heavily on procedure, I agree with many of Hill's points which I have verified through my own experimentation. Hill stated in one chapter that he had studied the lives of historical figures who possessed exceptional reasoning abilities. After extensive research, he conducted an experiment which proved the power of the dyslexic subconscious mind to achieve inspiration through pictorial thought processes.

Before going to bed at night, Mister Hill would close his eyes and image that he was sitting in a room with the people whose lives he had studied for the purpose of holding a conference. These people, who he referred to as his "invisible counselors", would sit around a table and Hill would present questions to the group for the members to answer. These invisible counselors would answer Hill's questions in accordance with the understanding of them which Hill had obtained as a result of his research into their lives. In this way, Hill allowed his subconscious mind to present him with inspiration pictorially through the use of these invisible counselors, much in the same manner that Einstein allowed his subconscious mind to solve mathematical equations pictorially through the creation of his "hunt".

As time passed, Hill continued to hold meetings with the invisible counselors and he claimed that each member developed individual traits and habits which would effect the group as a whole. Then, according to Hill, the invisible counselors developed the ability to carry on discourse among themselves independent of Hill's desires. It was at this point that Hill disbanded the group for fear that a continuation of these conferences would affect his perception of reality.

I present the example of Napoleon Hill and his invisible counselors to illustrate the power of the dyslexic subconscious mind and the vast potential which exists for each dyslexic if he is willing to explore his subconscious mind. It also presents an insight into the danger which exists for dyslexics if they reach a point where their alternate reality becomes as real as reality itself. This example explains one dyslexic phenomena which is rarely discussed and may cause embarrassment and confusion for dyslexics. The dyslexic may physically respond to alternate reality as though it were actual reality because both are experienced equally. As a result, a dyslexic may speak out loud if he imagines himself in a conversation even though he is completely alone. This tendency is difficult for the dyslexic to overcome and non-dyslexics should attempt to understand and accept the dyslexic's tendency to "think out loud".

Chapter Four
THE PHILOSOPHY OF BUREAUCRACY MANIPULATION

If we accept the definition of college as a preparatory experience
before entering the "real world", then dyslexics must develop
strategies to succeed in college, as well as life after college. For
this reason, it will be necessary for the dyslexic student to analyze
the college system in order to develop strategies to succeed.

A PREVIEW OF BUREAUCRACY

The first task in developing effective success strategies will be for
the dyslexic student to identify the various obstacles which will
likely be encountered in college in order to determine ways in which
to prevent them or to overcome them in the event that they may not be
avoided. Subsequent chapters will provide recommendations regarding
this process, however, at present, I will focus strictly on the
philosophical aspects of developing effective success strategies.
     The college, as any bureaucratic institution, operates based on
assumptions which are accepted as facts by the administration. In this
way, the administration attempts to control members of the
organization by anticipating the various ways in which they will
respond in the event of conflict and developing responses to these
actions which either protect the institution or discourage members
from taking action in the first place. The college strives to achieve
a high level of continuity with respect to policy and procedure,
therefore, any situation which arises to challenge either will be
treated as a threat to the system itself due to the possibility that
change could result.

Historically, dyslexic students have been treated as a threat to the continuity of college administrative policies because they require special accommodations on an individual basis due to the fact that no two cases of dyslexia may be treated equally. Therefore, colleges attempted to impose "standard treatment of dyslexia" policies which applied to all dyslexic students. Special treatment would have disrupted the systems' procedures due to this individual attention, so colleges attempted to protect themselves by imposing obstacles which would cause dyslexic students to fail.

Today, the chances of dyslexic students being victimized in college are unlikely due to the passage of the Americans With Disabilities Act which narrowly defines the rights of dyslexic students and the responsibilities of educational institutions to accommodate dyslexia. I will discuss this law and specific strategies for dealing with academic conflict in subsequent chapters. In this chapter, I will discuss the formulation of success strategies in theory as they pertain to bureaucratic systems under which the dyslexic is likely function during his life.

DEVELOPMENT OF THE BUREAUCRACY MANIPULATION PHILOSOPHY

A bureaucracy contains numerous flaws because it relies on procedures, it is inflexible, and it is resistant to change. The dyslexic has an inherent ability to pictorially analyze a bureaucracy in the same manner in which he may analyze a physical object to identify flaws. Once bureaucratic flaws have been identified, the dyslexic may find ways in which to not only avoid obstacles, but actually exploit the weaknesses which exist in the system to his best advantage. In order to do so, it will be necessary for the dyslexic to develop a personal philosophy to combat bureaucracy. This philosophy must accomplish several tasks in order for the dyslexic to succeed in the face of opposition.

First, the philosophy must safeguard the dyslexic against negative feelings of inferiority and helplessness. In order to accomplish this task, the dyslexic must view the bureaucracy from the point of view of a person who is not directly involved in its activities or affected by the decisions of its administration. This distance will place the dyslexic on the higher level of conscious awareness in which the subconscious mind may work efficiently to identify weaknesses within the bureaucracy which may be exploited.

Second, the philosophy must develop in such a way as to utilize the bureaucracy's rules and regulations. The dyslexic must either defeat the bureaucracy by identifying and manipulating inconsistencies in rules and regulations or endure procedures which have been implemented to combat opposition. The bureaucracy assumes that dyslexics will have two choices when faced with conflict: either to follow procedures which will not affect the continuity of the system, or to combat the system and face the consequences which have been established to protect against opposition. Either way, the bureaucracy is secure because its administration believes there to be little chance of significant opposition. This security is actually a weakness on which the dyslexic may capitalize because the administration will be unprepared to deal with an opponent who challenges their authority.

If the dyslexic identifies flaws in the system and combats the bureaucracy in accordance with established rules and regulations, then the system will be severely weakened because its procedures to combat opposition will be inadequate. In order to effectively react to success strategies which are based on system flaws, a bureaucracy must adopt new rules and regulations to prevent future opposition. This change will be difficult for the bureaucracy to enact. Therefore, the dyslexic's ability to negotiate a settlement with the administration will improve at this point due to the effort which the bureaucracy must expend in order to overcome its own flaws in the event that no acceptable resolution is found.

Third, the philosophy must convert disadvantages into advantages. The unique dyslexic ability to analyze not only the bureaucracy itself, but also the different groups which work within the bureaucracy and those which deal with the system from the outside, will enable the dyslexic to identify relations between these groups which may be beneficial in formulating a success strategy. The bureaucracy operates to the benefit of all members equally in theory while privately weeding out those members who it considers to be undesirable. The bureaucracy may consider the dyslexic to be undesirable due to his creative abilities and tendencies toward innovation which could result in change. The dyslexic must capitalize on the tendency of the bureaucracy to reject innovation in order to present a contradictory image of the bureaucracy to its members and outside groups.

The bureaucracy exists to promote change in theory, even though it may oppose change in practice. If the bureaucracy is seen to be oppressive to the dyslexic, questions will be raised regarding the reason. If members of the bureaucracy see that the system operates in conflict with its theorized purpose by combating an innovative dyslexic, the bureaucracy will appear to function in contradiction to its stated purpose and the competence of its leadership will questioned. The dyslexic must realize that an inverse relationship usually exists between the size of a bureaucratic system and the level of concern which each member holds for the bureaucracy. A large bureaucracy will employ thousands of members who consider themselves to be rather insignificant in relation to the grand purpose of the system. As a result, members often experience feelings of inadequacy and resentment toward the bureaucracy which the dyslexic may exploit to gain empathy with members who could eventually serve as allies in the event of conflict.

MAHATMA GHANDI AND THE END OF BRITISH RULE

In order to illustrate the three points of an effective success strategy, I will focus on one example in which these points were used to overcome bureaucratic opposition: the life of Mahatma Ghandi. Ghandi lived and worked in India during the first half of this century under the rule of the British Empire. Ghandi was without status or wealth, yet he developed a success strategy which was so effective that it enabled India to gain national independence from Britain.

One day, Mahatma Ghandi sat down. Although he was required to work, he protested British rule nonviolently by refusing to continue. By presenting himself as a challenge to the bureaucracy he was beaten and therefore suffered the consequences of procedures which the British colonial system had implemented to protect itself from opposition. The British government rationalized that physical assault would weaken opposition from the Indian people due to the fear that physical coercion would instill in those who would rebel. Ghandi, on

26

the other hand, understood that he could turn disadvantages into advantages, so the next day he returned to work and sat down. Again he was beaten. The next day, he sat down again. This cycle continued and others began to sit down. They were beaten. When they were released from prison, they returned to work, sat down, and others followed their example.

Eventually, Ghandi had such a following among the Indian people that the British Empire could no longer function economically in India. The British Empire lost its ability to control the Indian people because Ghandi had shown them how to take control of their own lives through the implementation of an effective success strategy. Physical coercion had empowered the British Empire for three hundred years until Ghandi showed the Indian people that his ability to withstand the beatings made him stronger than the British Empire which provided them. Ghandi defeated the British Empire by turning its source of control against the bureaucracy, thus deriving an advantage from what had previously been viewed as a great disadvantage. The British rule of India ended when the British government could no longer coerce the Indian people.

Ghandi succeeded in formulating a plan to combat the British Empire which incorporated all three components I have mentioned above. His plan identified and manipulated flaws in the British system, it worked within the system's parameters because he endured the procedures which the system had implemented to protect itself from opposition, and it turned disadvantages into advantages by showing that it takes more strength to endure a beating than it does to inflict one.

A PICTORIAL REPRESENTATION OF THE BUREAUCRACY MANIPULATION PHILOSOPHY

When conceiving of success strategies to defeat a bureaucratic system, it may benefit the dyslexic to pictorially visualize the developmental process of a star before it explodes as a "Great Nova". In the beginning, a star, such as our own sun, burns light gases such as hydrogen and helium by splitting atoms through high temperatures which are emitted from the movement of atomic particles which combine at the core to form more complex molecules. As the process continues, atomic particles collect to form elements which contain more complex atomic structures. These elements become increasing more complex and burn with ever-decreasing force due to the high level of heat which is absorbed to burn the more complex molecules. Eventually, the molecules combine to form iron, which is an element that absorbs, rather than emits, heat. The absorption of heat into the iron core causes the star's energy to implode into a tightly compressed mass until it can no longer be held together by gravity and violently explodes, blowing parts of the star throughout the galaxy.

A bureaucratic system establishes various responses to combat opposition just as a star burns various elements. The elements which a star burns become increasingly more complex until they can no longer be consumed. The responses enacted by a bureaucracy to combat opposition become increasingly more difficult to implement due to the fact that they increase in complexity as the opposition remains undefeated. These responses are based upon a least-common-denominator theory which states that the system may efficiently overcome most opposition through the expense of minimal effort. In order for the theory to work, potential opponents to the system must be willing to concede defeat as a result of the threat of retaliation, rather than

27

the implementation of these measures. If all potential opponents to the system were to accept these measures, the bureaucracy would be unable to expend the resources necessary to maintain such a conflict. The bureaucracy concedes defeat when it reaches the point where it can no longer respond to opposition just as a star will implode when it can no longer form elements which will emit heat.

BUREAUCRACY MANIPULATION AGAINST SUPERIOR OPPOSITION

I have developed a motto which I use to formulate success strategies when faced with bureaucratic opposition: "You must derive strength through weakness in order to obtain victory through defeat." This motto may seem contradictory at first, however, it is the basis for my philosophy of bureaucracy manipulation and very effective against opposition. In order to illustrate its effectiveness, I will provide one example in which my philosophy has proven successful in dealing with overwhelming bureaucratic opposition.

After I graduated from college in 1989, I pursued business opportunities in Siberia after participating in a cultural exchange between The University of Texas at Austin and Irkutsk State University. I traveled to the Irkutsk region in 1991 where I lived and worked until 1994. In 1992, I attempted to organize a program of economic cooperation between the State of Texas and the Irkutsk region by arranging contact between the governors of both states. The project failed due to corruption in the regional government and I was threatened by Siberian officials who wished to destroy my business by confiscating any containers of goods which I would import into or export out of the Irkutsk region.

In July 1993, a conspiracy was discovered and halted by a senior Siberian official in which members of the Irkutsk KGB and militia had filed a document which denounced me as a foreign spy in order to confiscate my property in Siberia and ensure that I could never return to Russia after I had left. I was informed at that time of a newspaper article which had been written that would have denounced me as a spy if the conspiracy had not been halted.

In January 1994, after forming a joint venture with a Siberian company and shipping a sea container of semi-precious stones to the Bratsk city railyard, a warrant was issued for my arrest and the container was impounded by the militia. I managed to evade a search which was conducted for me at all addresses where I had previously lived and I returned to Dallas on February 1.

At this point, I developed a success strategy to overcome bureaucratic opposition. My situation was dire and I realized that the process of overcoming bureaucratic opposition would be difficult for the following reasons: a) I was without assets due to the confiscation of my container, b) I had no legal protection in Russia and could not return due to the warrant which had been issued for my arrest in Bratsk, c) I could not prove that I had been victimized by corruption or even that the stones in the container were my property because my Russian partner had stolen all documents which pertained to the container and the joint venture. I contacted the appropriate American government agencies to make inquiries into this matter, however, there was little chance of resolution through official channels because I was without evidence to support my claims.

It was obvious that I could not defeat the Siberian officials who had destroyed my company, so I devised a plan under which they would defeat themselves. I formulated my success strategy by first assuming that I was not meant to leave the Irkutsk region alive and that the Siberian officials' plan to destroy my business had not anticipated my successful escape to America. I attempted to exploit this failure in the Siberians' plan by faxing condescending letters to the governor of the Irkutsk region, Yuri Nojikov, and the mayor of Bratsk, Ivan Nevmerzhitsky, which threatened to expose corruption on the part of regional officials if my property was not returned. I wrote the letters in such a way as to conflict with feelings of Russian nationalism and Siberian independence in order to exact a response. I believed that Siberian officials would either return my property at this point or denounce me for espionage, which had been the basis for the failed conspiracy in 1993.

In April and May, I was denounced in three Russian newspapers as a spy and smuggler by two generals in the FSK, the Russian Federation Counterintelligence Agency, which replaced the KGB after the fall of the Soviet Union. The articles even reported that I had been arrested and that my arrest constituted the greatest accomplishment of the Irkutsk FSK branch. Armed with these Russian articles, the U.S. Government had irrefutable evidence that I had been victimized by regional officials and my conflict was soon the subject of a syndicated American newspaper article. I faxed a copy of this article to mayor Nevmerzhitsky along with another letter in which I threatened to use the Russian articles to expose corruption which existed in the region to other American business people. In response, the Bratsk militia murdered the oldest son of my former partner and denounced me extensively in a four-part series of articles which appeared in regional newspapers. This time, I was reported to be an enemy of the Russian people and an idiot. After receiving copies of these Siberian articles, I arranged press coverage of my plight in three American business publications.

This conflict has lasted for sixteen months and I am now in a better position than ever to achieve resolution. A Russian customs inquiry is presently being conducted on the recommendation of the Russian trade representation office in Washington and senior officials in the Russian Ministry of Foreign Relations. My case has been reviewed by numerous American government agencies and I have examined American law thoroughly to develop a contingency plan to retaliate against Irkutsk officials in the event that official channels fail to provide an acceptable resolution. Although successful resolution of this conflict is not guaranteed, I may now expose corruption within the Irkutsk region which was virtually unknown to the world before my arrival in 1991.

ANALYSIS AND MANIPULATION OF A CORRUPT BUREAUCRACY

The weaknesses in the Irkutsk bureaucracy were the following: 1) Irkutsk officials considered their actions to be absolute due to the power they had enjoyed under the former Soviet system. 2) They were unaware that actions taken against me in Bratsk could have an international effect because they had previously been isolated from the world. 3) They failed to understand the concept of representative democracy and assumed that I would have no representation in the American government due to the fact that I am a small businessman. 4) They failed to realize that the procedures which their system had used to protect itself from opposition in the past could strengthen, rather than weaken, a citizen of a foreign country. 5) They believed unquestionably in their own invincibility. 6) Their system relied on a rigid hierarchy.

In order to succeed in this conflict, I had to obtain evidence of persecution from Irkutsk officials in order to manipulate the weaknesses of their system. They provided this evidence through their attempts to protect themselves against retaliatory measures I might take in America. They relentlessly denounced me in the Russian press because this was the means by which they had historically weakened opposition. In reality, these actions strengthened me and secured a position from which I could retaliate against them.

In the early stages of this conflict, I opposed regional officials who could have resolved this conflict easily by returning the stones. By denouncing me in the Russian press, they escalated the conflict and I retaliated by threatening to expose corruption in high levels of the regional government to the American press. They responded by denouncing me again and committing murder in an attempt to protect themselves from investigations which could result from my claims regarding corruption on their part. I responded to the denunciations by threatening to take action against the national government of Russia in the American press under the provisions of the U.S. Constitution and Bill of Rights and demanding ten million dollars compensation from the Russian government for human rights violations which Irkutsk officials had committed against me. It was at this point that the National Russian Government intervened to investigate the matter.

I viewed my conflict in terms of military strategy in order to devise my plan to overcome bureaucratic opposition. While in Siberia, I fought a defensive battle on foreign soil, with limited resources, among people who I couldn't trust, based on information I couldn't believe, in order to transport a container of stones which I had to protect. A Siberian associate once called mine a "no exit situation". When my container was confiscated by Irktusk officials, I was strengthened because I had reached a point from which I had nothing left to lose. In America, vast amounts of information were at my disposal, I was provided resources as an American citizen through government agencies, and I was in an offensive, rather than defensive, position from which I would act and Irkutsk officials react, rather than the reverse. In essence, by confiscating my container, Irkutsk officials had provided me with an exit.

In order to exploit the Russian system of hierarchy, I proceeded with a plan of escalation while, at the same time, provided Irkutsk officials the means to resolve the conflict at every point. Every time the conflict escalated, a higher Russian office became involved which chose to protect subordinates rather than negotiate to resolve the conflict. Also, with each escalation, the potential loss sustainable by Irkutsk officials increased. What had begun as an attempt to destroy my company had blossomed into an international incident which could destroy the reputation of the Irkutsk region, thus restricting badly needed foreign investment while increasing the chance for internal investigation of regional officials.

The ability of Irkutsk officials to quickly resolve the matter diminished due to my demand for compensation as a result of human rights violations. With every escalation, the pressure which subordinate Russian agencies experienced from their superiors increased due to their involvement in a conflict for which they were not responsible and under which they could conceivably sustain damage as participants. The hierarchical stress which results from my strategy of escalation serves to weaken and divide the opposition until the Russian hierarchy realizes that it can no longer protect

Irkutsk officials and their superiors will intervene to resolve the conflict.

I also followed an escalation strategy when dealing with American officials to resolve this conflict. I began by working with the Commerce and State Departments and then expanded my efforts to question the actions of the U.S. Congress in granting economic aid to Russia in view of my conflict. I determined that the granting of economic aid to Russia without the existence of legal protection for American citizens in Russia violates the constitutional rights of the American taxpayers. In this way, the blame for this incident may also be placed on the actions of the U.S. Government in the event that no resolution is found by appealing to the voters who elected the officials who have decided to aid Russia.

The conflict which I am experiencing with Irkutsk officials is not yet resolved, however, I have managed to significantly improve my position in this conflict through the formulation and implementation of a success strategy which has accomplished the three tasks which are required to combat bureaucratic opposition. At this point, it seems unlikely that the conflict will remain unresolved due to the attention which this matter has received from officials within the American and Russian governments. Irkutsk officials are now aware that failure to resolve this conflict will not result in its termination, but rather, its escalation.

In this chapter, I have attempted to demonstrate the theoretical processes which the dyslexic may use to develop success strategies in order to overcome bureaucratic opposition. The examples which have been provided should illustrate the proper usage of success strategies and demonstrate their effectiveness. The information which has been presented in this and previous chapters serves as a preview to the information which is contained in subsequent chapters. The remainder of this book will be an exercise in the practical application of these theories.

Chapter Five
SUCCESS BEGINS IN HIGH SCHOOL

Now that we have discussed the various components of dyslexia and theories for formulating success strategies, the time has come to apply this information to real life experiences. To begin this segment, I will focus on the high school experience in order to provide a preview into the more detailed subject of college.

THE DYSLEXIC HIGH SCHOOL STUDENT

By the time the dyslexic student reaches high school, he should have already adopted several success strategies which he has frequently used to overcome obstacles in grade school. Much of the information which he uses to formulate these strategies exists on a subconscious level, therefore, he is unaware of the cognitive processes which are involved to incorporate it into his strategies. The remainder exists on a conscious level. He uses this information to formulate success strategies based on positive experiences from the past.

High school is most significant because performance during this time will determine the dyslexic student's options for college. In turn, the college which he attends will determine his career options after graduation. This relationship illustrates the importance of succeeding in high school because high school performance directly affects the future.

The dyslexic high school student must work within greater confines than the dyslexic college student because he has less control over the courses he must take and he must function within the public school system, which is often comprised of teachers and administrators who do not understand dyslexia or know how to deal with it. It is for these reasons that the dyslexic high school student must formulate effective strategies to succeed in high school.

The advantage of high school over college is that high school course work is less extensive and easier to comprehend than that of college. This difference exists because the high school prepares students to function in society after graduation, however, not all high school students will seek further education and will instead enter the workforce. For these students, comprehension of college level material is not required.

THE DYSLEXIC STUDENT AND LEGAL REPRESENTATION

Before I continue, I would like to point out that the dyslexic student currently enjoys more rights and protection under American law than at any time in history. Only five years ago, the common practice among administrators, in both high school and college, was to require dyslexic students to complete course work for which they had never received adequate instruction. In this way, the responsibility for accommodating dyslexia fell on the dyslexic student and his family rather than the school administration. At the time, the only law which existed to protect the dyslexic student was Section 504 of The Vocational Rehabilitation Act of 1974 which guaranteed that schools would make "reasonable accommodation" for dyslexic students. This law had been extensively tested in court and weakened to the point where it provided virtually no legal protection to dyslexic students.

The Vocational Rehabilitation Act was flawed because dyslexia was not well understood in 1974, so abstract terms were used to describe accommodations which schools were required to implement for dyslexic students. It was assumed that standard methods of treatment would be discovered and implemented once they had been identified. To the contrary, research into dyslexia proved that no two cases are identical because each dyslexic reacts differently to his environment and develops means to deal with the inconsistencies which he perceives.

The situation faced by dyslexic students in American schools was extremely repressive because they had to perform in a system which taught in a verbal/linear fashion while experiencing thought pictorially. A common belief among administrators and teachers at that time was that dyslexia was a form of laziness and to accommodate such a condition would in effect reinforce tendencies which they considered to be counter-productive. This position was justified by reasoning that any accommodations made in course work would weaken the school's image due to the dyslexic student's ability to graduate without having completed the established academic requirements.

The dyslexic student was often subjected to ridicule by school officials when requesting accommodations and frequently failed to satisfactorily complete required course work. As a result, he would often suffer from a negative self-image due to the high school's refusal to provide accommodations which were guaranteed by law.

On July 26, 1990, the Americans With Disabilities Act was passed into law by congress. It eliminated all ambiguity which existed with respect to accommodating dyslexia, not only in schools but also in the business community.

Fortunately, a legal framework finally exists to protect the dyslexic student. It should no longer be necessary for the dyslexic student to fight a hostile school bureaucracy in order to receive accommodations, however, it is the dyslexic student's responsibility to create an environment under which the school may best serve his needs.

METHODS TO OBTAIN ACCOMMODATIONS IN HIGH SCHOOL

The first step to receiving accommodations in high school is to obtain documentation from a reputable physician which verifies the existence of dyslexia. This documentation should include any available test results as well as a letter from the physician which summarizes the condition and requests that accommodations be made.

Once documentation is in order, The dyslexic student should request a conference between the high school principal and his parents to discuss the various accommodations which will be required. This meeting will serve not only to avoid complications in the future with respect to accommodations, but will inform the high school administration of the dyslexic student's needs. It should also prove useful in forming a relationship with the principal which may be utilized in the future when seeking further accommodations. Under the provisions of the Americans With Disabilities Act, the principal cannot refuse to grant accommodations. However, if the principal is reluctant to make accommodations after documentation has been received, the dyslexic student should inform him that the matter will be discussed with his superiors if he is unwilling to cooperate.

Once accommodations have been granted, the dyslexic student should contact the nearest office of his State Rehabilitation Commission (the Rehab) to be registered as a member in order to receive any benefits which their offices provide in accordance with various state and federal programs. The Rehab also provides assistance in the resolution of academic conflict. In the event that conflict should arise during the high school years which the administration is either unwilling or unable to resolve, the Rehab may appoint a case worker to represent the dyslexic student as advocate in order to resolve the matter. He may also contact the state Commission For The Blind which offers benefits to dyslexics. Their legal department may intervene to resolve the conflict if the dyslexic student feels that this action would be beneficial.

I present this information based on past experiences rather than an anticipation of events which are likely to occur. The new legal protection which exists for dyslexics reduces the likelihood that conflict will arise which the high school administration will be unable to resolve. Conflict is also unlikely because the high school is a bureaucratic institution in which administrators would be unwilling to place themselves in a difficult position by denying accommodations which would ultimately be the teacher's responsibility to carry out.

THE FORMULATION OF HIGH SCHOOL SUCCESS STRATEGIES

Once accommodations have been identified and implemented by the high school administration, the dyslexic student must formulate success strategies which will allow him to graduate in four years with a high grade-point-average (GPA). The ability to conceive and implement high school success strategies will serve as practice for college where such strategic planning will be crucial to academic survival.

Before formulating success strategies, the dyslexic student must obtain information regarding the high school in order to obtain a base of knowledge from which to work. He must identify all sources of assistance which will be available and use these sources to his advantage. He must analyze the academic requirements which must be satisfied in order to graduate and identify ways in which he may complete this work with the least amount of effort. He should also know if he may advance directly to higher classes if his abilities warrant such a move and analyze the procedures which would allow him to do so. In this way, he may avoid classes which are beneath his academic level and allow him to focus attention on subjects which will be more useful in college. An effective success strategy which utilizes the option to advance to higher classes will allow the dyslexic student to graduate in less than the standard four years.

The first task in formulating an effective success strategy will be for the dyslexic student to identify people who may assist in his pursuit of information. These people may be administrators or teachers, however, he should cultivate relationships with them which he may utilize throughout the high school years to overcome difficult situations. If the dyslexic student has developed his natural ability to see the world through another's eyes, he may use this ability to endear himself to people within the high school from whom he may obtain the greatest advantage.

This "information group" will greatly assist the dyslexic student throughout the high school years if he succeeds in conveying himself positively to them because the knowledge and influence of each member will increase his capability to overcome bureaucratic opposition from the high school administration. Although the high school is governed by a system of rules and procedures in theory, it operates to a great extent upon the perceptions which school officials hold of individual students. If the dyslexic student is perceived to be intelligent by his information group, he will be expected to perform well. As a result, he may avoid harsh criticism in situations which may require it due to the influence which the members of his information group hold over people who would create obstacles for him.

The second task in formulating an effective success strategy will be to identify people within the high school who the dyslexic student believes will obstruct his ability to succeed. For whatever reason, there are usually people within high school administrations who do not approve of dyslexics and they often create obstacles which dyslexic students must overcome. The information group should assist the dyslexic student in locating classes which are taught by teachers who understand his needs, however, he should also talk to fellow students to identify teachers who are naturally obstructive. If these people may be identified, the dyslexic student may avoid difficult situations which they may cause.

THE DYSLEXIC STUDENT AND THE MANIPULATION OF HIGH SCHOOL POLITICS

Success in high school will depend as much upon the dyslexic student's ability to receive and comprehend information regarding school politics and current events than it will on his understanding of high school course work. After the high school system is analyzed, the dyslexic student should realize that the high school places little emphasis on his ability to learn the required material, but rather, on his ability to perform rote processes which are designed to suggest that he understands this material. I will discuss methods which may be used to improve GPA in later chapters, however, I will now focus on the interpersonal aspects of succeeding in high school by providing examples from my own experiences.

The dyslexic student must realize that the high school does not identify actual intelligence in students, but rather, perceived intelligence which is evaluated by individual teachers. For this reason, the ability of a dyslexic student to convey an intelligent image of himself will positively effect the grade which he receives in high school classes. The process of developing beneficial interpersonal relationships with teachers provides valuable practice for success in college and beyond.

I attended the Business and Management Center High School (BMC) in Dallas from 1981 to 1984. The American education system's reputation was dismal during my high school years due to high levels of bureaucracy and the inability to attract qualified teachers. At the time, the Texas education system ranked forty-eighth in the nation while The Dallas Independent School District was ranked as one of the poorest districts in Texas with respect to overall academic performance.

I arrived at BMC in the Fall of 1981 after having spent six years in private schools which claimed to treat dyslexia. I had not attended public school since the third grade, during which time I had received instruction in special classes which taught language comprehension to a greater degree than those offered by the public school system. The other students had already completed the Spring semester, so I had to complete this work while attending classes during the Fall semester. I quickly realized the difference in education levels between public and private schools when I reviewed the required course work for the Spring semester because the level of difficulty was considerably lower than that to which I was accustomed. I required two weeks to complete all course work from the Spring semester and I finished my freshman year on the outstanding students' list.

During the Fall semester, I analyzed the high school bureaucracy and identified flaws in the system which would benefit me academically. One major flaw was that the teachers' pay raises were linked to the students' performance on biannual examinations which were administered by the Texas Education Association to determine the average level of student academic comprehension. The teachers were given copies of these tests for review along with answer sheets which they used to evaluate student performance on mock tests which were administered prior to the actual exam.

The examination system was flawed because it gave the teachers and the students a mutual interest in the achievement of high test scores. As a result, it was not uncommon for teachers to provide answers on the mock tests which would allow the students to correctly answer questions which would be asked on the actual exam. In this way, the students would receive high exam scores which did not adequately reflect their knowledge of the subjects tested and the teachers benefited financially when the results of the exam reflected a substantial improvement from the previous semester.

This procedure set a precedent which was potentially beneficial to students during class. If the answers to biannual exam questions were made available to students without instruction, then the same process should have existed to a certain degree with regard to material which was taught in class. Otherwise, an inconsistency in procedure could have resulted which would have suggested that a double standard existed. I managed to utilize this inconsistency in class during my second semester to obtain previews to course work which I doubt that I would have otherwise received.

I utilized this inconsistency for three semesters until a group of teachers from another high school were discovered revealing copies of biannual exams to students in an attempt to improve overall performance. The testing procedure was quickly modified to prevent teachers from manipulating the testing process. Afterward, The State Board of Education required teachers in Texas to take exams which evaluated their academic comprehension. After fierce opposition, the exam was administered and the results showed that the teachers themselves had only a mediocre comprehension of the subjects which they taught. Under such conditions, my high school bureaucracy was easy to manipulate, given correct information on a timely basis.

It was also not uncommon in my high school for courses to end before the required material had been completed. In one class, the students never progressed beyond the third chapter in the course textbook. In another class, the teacher had suffered a recent divorce which had left her emotionally distraught. Instead of completing the required course work, the students spent class periods counseling the teacher on her personal life and barely understood the required material for the course. The best grades in this class were given to students who offered the most useful advice. I was particularly active in this class and received an "A" for my efforts.

The most productive success strategy which I formulated during my high school years was implemented during the junior year when I participated in an internship program. The program allowed students to work at a job during the fifth, sixth, and seventh periods in order to receive experience in the workplace rather than classroom instruction. The grade for the internship program was based on performance evaluations which the school provided to the students' employers. At the end of each pay period, the students would report the wages which they had earned to the internship coordinator and the school district would then receive ten percent of this amount from the state education operations fund.

In the beginning, I worked as a salesman in a shoe store until I was laid-off due to poor company earning. At the time, the internship coordinator was hospitalized after having undergone heart surgery. His replacement showed no interest in the program and never attended the weekly meetings during which the interns would discuss their progress. As I had no classes in the afternoon, I went home every day and worked at a salvage business which I had operated since 1974. Instead of selling shoes, I would spend my afternoons collecting scrap metal at construction sites and dealing in used machinery. After several weeks, I contacted a member of my information group who allowed me to register my salvage business as an internship. What the high school administration failed to realize, however, was that I was without an employer as an entrepreneur. As such, I filled out my own student evaluation forms and gave myself excellent grades for my outstanding performance in the salvage business.

During my high school years, I was unaware of my legal rights to receive academic accommodations for dyslexia and none were provided. Nevertheless, I graduated from high school with a 3.20 GPA and placed fourteenth out of a class of 212. My success was not due to the ability to conform to verbal/linear thought processes, but rather, to the low academic requirements which the high school placed on students coupled with my ability to effect change and manipulate the high school bureaucracy. I regret that my high school years were not more educational, however, I received practical experience in the formulation and implementation of effective success strategies. This knowledge would be instrumental to my performance at college during the following years.

THE DYSLEXIC STUDENT AND THE SCHOLASTIC ASSESSMENT TEST

The final challenge from high school comes in the form of the SAT (Scholastic Assessment Test) which evaluates the student's comprehension of the subjects which he should have been taught in high school. If the student graduates in the top ten percent of his class, his scores on the SAT will not be considered by college admissions offices when determining entrance eligibility. The dyslexic student is entitled to take the SAT untimed under conditions which do not conflict with his dyslexia. In order to avoid complications, he must contact the person who will administer the SAT and personally verify that the necessary accommodations will be made rather than rely on high school counselors or administrators to organize accommodations. These people may not understand what accommodations must be made or they may not act at all if there has previously been conflict between the dyslexic student and the high school administration.

If the dyslexic student feels that he will experience difficulty with the material on the SAT, he must contact the high school administration and arrange a tutor to assist in studying for the test. Because the SAT is given during the senior year, the dyslexic student will have ample time to prepare for the test should he wish to begin studying early. The assistance offered by a tutor is valuable for the dyslexic student because the interaction between the two may provide a positive learning environment if mutual relations are good.

The dyslexic student must decide whether to take the SAT with or without accommodations. Under The Americans With Disabilities Act, State colleges are required to pay all expenses involved in the education of dyslexic students, however, private colleges may refuse to admit dyslexic applicants on this basis because they would lose money if the cost of accommodations exceeded the tuition paid by the dyslexic student. If the dyslexic student plans to attend a private college, he may wish to take the SAT timed if he has earned a high GPA in high school or if he has finished in the top ten percent of his graduating class. If the dyslexic student takes the SAT timed, he is not required under law to identify himself as dyslexic when applying to a private college. If the private college admits the dyslexic applicant, he may later identify himself as dyslexic and the private college will be bound by law to pay for all accommodations he will require for the time he attends the private college.

Chapter Six
ENTERING COLLEGE

Before high school graduation, the dyslexic student must determine which college will be most suitable and apply for admission. The various factors which must be taken into consideration when choosing a college are the quality of academic programs offered by the college, tuition & expenses, geographic location, and type of institution.

The high school will prepare a transcript of the classes which have been completed and submit it to the admissions offices of the colleges to which the dyslexic student wishes to apply. These colleges must be compared for the dyslexic student to determine what course of study, or major, will best suit his career goals and then apply for admission.

The two types of colleges are state and private. State colleges will benefit the dyslexic student if his academic performance in high school meets their entrance requirements because they must provide and pay for all accommodations which he will require during the time he attends the college. State colleges are funded by tax dollars and may not discriminate against applicants on the basis of dyslexia. Private colleges, on the other hand, are not federally funded and may reject dyslexic applicants due to legal requirements for them to pay for accommodations. This added expense might be viewed as being economically unfeasible by the private college administration and discriminatory policies could be in place to prevent the enrollment of dyslexic students.

Prior to applying for admissions to a private college, the dyslexic applicant should request a copy of the college's admissions policy to determine if the college has implemented exclusion policies which would result in the rejection of his admissions application. If the dyslexic applicant wishes to attend a private college, but does not wish to identify himself as dyslexic, he may legally do so and the private college will be required to provide and pay for all accommodations he will require during the time he attends the college if his admissions application is accepted.

Regardless of the college to which the dyslexic applicant wishes to apply, he should analyze the various scholarships which may be available to him if he has performed well in high school. Public libraries offer books which list scholarships that are available to high school graduates along with the stipulations which accompany them. Although the process of applying for scholarships often seems confusing to the college applicant, an afternoon in a public library should provide all information needed to evaluate what, if any, scholarship options exist.

It will also be beneficial for the dyslexic applicant to contact the Rehab to determine if any state funded programs exist to pay college tuition expenses for dyslexic students. When I attended The University of Texas at Austin, the Rehab provided payment of college tuition up to $450 per semester. The Rehab paid this amount directly to the university upon receipt of course acceptance confirmations. The Rehab should be contacted as soon as the college admissions application has been approved to determine if financial aid is available.

When responses arrive regarding admissions applications, the dyslexic student should visit the various colleges which he has chosen to determine how they will suit him personally. He may be required to move to another city if the campus is located far from his home or he may wish to attend a local college. Colleges hold visitors' days prior to the beginning of each semester when applicants may compare the programs and facilities offered by the college to those which are offered by other colleges. All colleges assist applicants in making informed admissions choices because an applicant who regrets his decision to attend a college will be discontent and may exhibit poor academic performance as a result.

Once the benefits and disadvantages of various colleges have been weighed, the dyslexic student must choose one and then make plans for the first semester. At this point, he should know whether or not he is eligible to receive economic aid or scholarships. He should also be familiar with the resources which the college offers and have a plan regarding the courses to which he will apply for the first semester.

Chapter Seven
PREPARING FOR THE FIRST SEMESTER

Once the dyslexic student has been admitted into college and is aware of available resources, he must choose the courses which he will take during the first semester. At this point he must develop a set of priorities and an image of himself in relation to the college. College can be a strange and impersonal place for a new student, especially if it is part of a large university.

THE DYSLEXIC STUDENT IN RELATION TO COLLEGE

The dyslexic student must realize that he alone is responsible for his performance at college. He must strive to succeed because it is what he wishes and not because academic success conforms to the wishes of friends and family. He will spend at least four years in college to earn a diploma. He will have difficulty with course work and/or professors and administrators, therefore, he will not succeed in college unless he has a strong desire to do so.

This strong desire to succeed must be accompanied by a realization that the college, and everyone who is employed by the college, exists to serve his needs. At this point, congratulations are in order because he has performed well enough in high school to enter college. He is now among the best and has been provided a college which contains resources sufficient to achieve his goals. From this point forward, he will work on his own initiative with the government providing financial, academic, and legal support.

THE DYSLEXIC STUDENT AND THE FORMULATION OF COLLEGE SUCCESS STRATEGIES

With the road to the future lying ahead, the dyslexic student must set priorities and formulate success strategies through which he will excel in college. He will have the choice of many courses that may be taken to fulfill academic requirements. He must determine whether he will take college courses to learn new subjects or to increase knowledge of subjects in which he already possesses significant knowledge.

In my opinion, it is better to take courses in areas in which significant knowledge already exists for the following reasons: First, specialized knowledge may be developed by concentrating study on one subject. This specialized knowledge will be beneficial later in life if the dyslexic decides to change careers. The major will only account for about half of the hours which must be completed in order to graduate, so the opportunity exists to gain extensive knowledge of a subject that is different from the major while satisfying requirements in other subjects. Second, grades improve if courses are taken which cover the same subject from different perspectives because the material is familiar. Third, study time is reduced because knowledge may be applied from previous courses which have covered the same material.

I met many students in college who enrolled in diverse, complicated courses in order to "expand their horizons." These courses required excessive study time, or specialized knowledge of the subject, in order to receive favorable grades. Many of the students who took these courses either failed or dropped out of college due to poor academic performance. Their horizons now stretch as far as the eye can see because they wasted their chance to succeed in college and have the rest of their lives to search for a career without a college diploma.

The dyslexic student should focus attention on courses which teach subjects that are pertinent to his career goals, or courses which teach subjects that are related to his major. The world is full of people who possess general knowledge which they never use. Careers which are available to college graduates demand specialized knowledge, therefore, graduates who have obtained general knowledge will not likely meet the requirements for these careers. If a college course teaches a subject of interest, but has a reputation for being difficult, the dyslexic student may obtain significant knowledge of the subject without enrolling in the course. The course textbook may be purchased and read during leisure time, or research of the subject may be done at college and public libraries. Resources are available to research any subject of interest without enrolling in a course which will risk the GPA.

Before registering for the first semester's courses, the dyslexic student should know if the college offers any placement tests on subjects in which he already possesses significant knowledge. If so, the dyslexic student should contact the director of the testing center to administer the placement test(s) under conditions which accommodate his dyslexia. He should also notify the Rehab of his intention to take placement test(s) because the funds which pay his tuition may also pay the fees for these tests. If the placement test is successfully completed, college credit is earned without having to enroll in a course which teaches the subject. I especially recommend placement tests to dyslexic students who speak foreign languages because a maximum 16 hours of college credit may be earned for each language. If placement tests are used to assess proficiency in foreign languages, it is possible for the dyslexic student who speaks a second language to advance to the sophomore year during the first semester.

The dyslexic student should not register for more than the average number of courses during the first semester because he will not know how well he will perform in college. Dyslexic students often work slower than non-dyslexic students and are unable to enroll in even the average number of courses. The dyslexic student will know within a couple of weeks after the semester begins whether or not he falls into this category by the amount of time which is required to study course material. The dyslexic student should not be concerned if time does not exist to adequately study course material. Colleges normally allow a month for students to drop courses and, if necessary, may extend this deadline if a dyslexic student feels that he cannot function because he is overloaded with course work.

Many colleges have a minimum number of credit hours which a student must take to receive full-time status. If his courses fall below this number, the dyslexic student should contact the college dean and obtain written permission to maintain full-time status while taking less than the required number of hours. The granting of full-time status to dyslexics who take less than the required number of credit hours is a normal accommodation for dyslexia.

A good strategy for the first year of college is to take an average, or slightly less than average, number of courses and study for placement tests during spare time. Placement tests may be taken untimed, so the director of the testing center should arrange a time and place for the placement test to be administered which conforms to the dyslexic student's schedule. If successful, the dyslexic student will have as many, or more, credit hours completed at the end of the first year than the student who took the average number of courses.

THE PLANNING OF AN EFFECTIVE ACADEMIC SCHEDULE

When planning academic schedules, the dyslexic student must evaluate his biological cycles in order to determine what times will be preferable to attend classes. When I attended college, I never registered for classes which began earlier than 10:00 AM and always allowed at least one hour for lunch. I occasionally missed the chance to take courses which would have suited my academic plan due to the fact that they conflicted with my biological cycles. I never strayed from my academic plan because I knew that I would not be receptive in the morning due to the fact that I experienced insomnia during college, and also because I would not be receptive to lectures if I had not been given sufficient time to eat lunch. Understanding biological cycles allowed me to plan my academic schedule in a manner which maintained harmony in my daily routine through which academic performance was facilitated.

CHOOSING THE CORRECT PROFESSORS

Once the dyslexic student has determined what courses and placement tests (if any) to take, he must notify the professors who will teach these courses of the accommodations which must be made and learn what requirements they place upon students who enroll in their courses. Most professors are understanding and willing to help dyslexic students, however, some will not. In this case, it is best to find another course in which to enroll, or enroll in the same course if it is taught by another professor who is receptive to accommodate dyslexia. Alternate courses are usually available which fulfill the same academic requirements of courses which are taught by professors with whom conflict is anticipated. The process of enrolling in an alternate course may be time consuming, however, it is far better to enroll in an alternate course which is taught by an understanding professor than to do poorly in a course in which accommodations are not granted and have a low grade appear permanently on the academic record as a result.

Occasionally, a professor will structure his course in a manner that conflicts with dyslexia and the dyslexic student's performance will be impaired as a result. If the dyslexic student feels he will experience difficulty as a result of course work, or that the course will consume too much spare time, he should seek other courses. If none are available, he must explain to the professor how and why the course will conflict with dyslexia as well as the accommodations which must be made to improve his comprehension of the subject.

If a conflict arises between a dyslexic student and a professor, the college dean must immediately be notified and a request must be made for his assistance to resolve the matter. An immediate request gives the situation a sense of urgency and demonstrates the dyslexic student's willingness to solve academic problems through administrative channels.

Chapter Eight
REDUCE WORK TIME AND IMPROVE GRADES

During the first semester, the dyslexic student will be required to complete many time-consuming assignments, so it will be necessary to reduce work time.

WORK TIME REDUCTION THROUGH TEXTBOOK SELECTION

The first step to reduce work time will be to obtain used, highlighted textbooks for college courses. Several used copies of each textbook should be selected and the highlighted text analyzed. Textbooks should be purchased in which the highlighted text presents a clear and concise message. The process of choosing well highlighted textbooks requires extra effort, but this time will have been well spent when textbooks have been purchased in which the most useful information is highlighted on text which represents only a fraction of the print. Textbook authors report subjects in far more detail than will be required for college courses because an average exam only covers the main points in a textbook.

In some cases, used textbooks will not be available, however, earlier editions of the textbook may be borrowed from the college library and compared to the new edition. Any significant changes should be noted which have been added to the new edition and the previous edition should be used to study for the course. The dyslexic student should not make the mistake of believing that he will do poorly in a college course by studying the previous edition of a new textbook. It is a common practice among textbook authors to make cosmetic changes to their textbooks in order to print new editions and market them for use in college courses.

Occasionally, new textbooks must be selected which will be categorized as either "recommended" or "required". Recommended textbooks should never be purchased from a college bookstore for use in a college course. A recommended textbook contains an in-depth analysis of the course subject, but the material contained within will not be covered on exams. If it were, the textbook would be required. Recommended textbooks should be borrowed from the college or public library only if the information is of interest to the dyslexic student. If no copy is available from libraries, a copy may be purchased from a wholesale bookstore. College bookstores often charge twice to three times the wholesale price for most textbooks.

Required new textbooks must be purchased from a college bookstore at the bookstore's price, but the dyslexic student need not spend time reading it from cover to cover. Instead, the disabled students' association should be contacted along with a request that a volunteer be assigned to read and highlight the new textbook. Once the textbook has been highlighted, the highlighted print may be studied when preparing for exams. The dyslexic student must never assume that he will fail or do poorly on exams if he does not study all information contained in the textbook. A well highlighted textbook will contain 90% of the information required for an exam on 10% of the text. If every word in a textbook is read, the dyslexic student will have so much information memorized at the time of the exam that he will be fortunate if he retains enough useful information to make a "C". The dyslexic student must always remember that he is in college to learn and to make good grades. The only way to do so is to focus on that which is important to ignore that which is not.

WORK TIME REDUCTION THROUGH GOVERNMENT SERVICES

Another option available to reduce work time is services offered by The Commission For The Blind. These services may be utilized by dyslexic students because dyslexia causes the inversion of letters and numbers when they read and write. Among these services is an extensive cassette tape library which is operated by a division of the Library of Congress called Reading For The Blind. Rather than having to read textbooks, the dyslexic student may borrow cassette tapes on which his textbooks have been recorded from which to study. If a cassette copy of the textbook has not previously been recorded, the printed textbook may be presented to Recording For The Blind and they will record it on cassette tape. They may also provide a variable-speed tape player on which to listen to these tapes at no charge.

WORK TIME REDUCTION THROUGH PASS/FAIL COURSES

Colleges often allow students to take a certain number of credit hours on a pass/fail basis, which means that college credit is received for a course without a grade. This option is beneficial if the dyslexic student has previously made good grades because it allows him to enroll in a course, make the lowest acceptable grade, and receive credit without lowering his GPA. A good success strategy is to take a course on a pass/fail basis during semesters when enrollment in difficult courses is unavoidable because more study time may be devoted to the difficult courses and less study time devoted to the

46

course which is taken on a pass/fail basis. If the dyslexic student has a low GPA, a good success strategy is to take courses which fulfill college requirements, but have a reputation for being easy. If he makes good grades in these courses, his GPA will rise and he may then take courses on a pass/fail basis to maintain it. It becomes more difficult to raise the GPA as the number of completed college credit hours increases because each course will subsequently represent a smaller percentage of the total completed credit hours.

WORK TIME REDUCTION THROUGH COMMUNITY COLLEGE SUMMER COURSES

The dyslexic student may also have the option to take courses at a community college during summers and transfer the credit hours to be applied toward his major. Taking summer courses at a community college is a good success strategy if the dyslexic student has performed well in college because the credit received will not affect his GPA. Courses which are taught at community colleges are usually easier than those taught at state or private colleges, so they offer the opportunity to receive college credit without having to do college level work.

   Colleges maintain lists of community college courses which fulfill degree requirements. When the dyslexic student checks this list for possible community college courses, he should see if any are offered on subjects which he has already studied. If so, these courses should be taken on a self-paced basis in which exams must be completed without attending a class. Many self-paced community college summer courses last for 5-1/2 weeks and require students to take multiple choice exams.

   When the textbook and study guide are purchased for the self-paced community college course, the information should be closely examined to determine if it has previously been covered in another course. If so, the study guide should be purchased without the textbook and notes from previous courses used when studying for exams. I took two 5-1/2 week self-paced courses at Austin Community College using this technique. I completed each in less than ten days and answered 85% of the exam question correctly in both courses.

   The dyslexic student must never register for a course at a community college unless he is certain that the credit will transfer and count toward his major. The dyslexic student must always contact the college dean when planning to take a community college course to determine if restrictions exist of which he is unaware. Finally, he must never register for summer school at his college unless he is certain that he will be able to complete 16 weeks of college course work during a 5-1/2 week semester.

ACADEMIC SUCCESS THROUGH THE DEVELOPMENT OF POSITIVE RELATIONSHIPS

Successfully reducing work time is vital to succeeding in college, however, it is also vital to develop positive relationships with professors because they are invaluable sources of information and they ultimately determine grades. The dyslexic student may begin to develop positive relationships with professors during first meetings to discuss course work and accommodations for dyslexia. Their assistance should be requested when clarification is required for information received in class and their office hours utilized to discuss impending assignments. This contact will show the professors that the dyslexic student is determined to learn and they will often go to great lengths to assist him. In addition, frequent visits should cause the dyslexic student and the professor to develop a mutual respect which will provide an advantage over other students who never contacted the professor. Although frequent contact is important, this time must be used to discuss subjects which are related to the course. Time spent socializing with the professor might be misinterpreted as an attempt to win favor rather than learn the course material. In this case, time spent with the professor could produce undesirable results.

Chapter Nine
MAKING THE MOST OF EXAMS

The ultimate determinant of success in college is the exam. Although
students may be tested in a number of ways, the four most common types
of exams are multiple choice, true/false, short answer, and essay. Any
of these may cause problems for a dyslexic student, so he should be
aware of the types of exams which cause the greatest difficulty. When
expected to take an exam which is structured in a manner that
conflicts with dyslexia, the dyslexic student should contact the
professor and request that the exam be administered in a manner which
accommodates dyslexia. The college is obligated by law to provide
accommodations for dyslexic students, so exams must be administered in
a manner which accurately tests comprehension on an untimed basis.

THE DEVELOPMENT OF EFFECTIVE STUDY METHODS

In order to succeed during exams, an effective method of study must be
found. During college, I would prepare for exams at least one week in
advance by studying for short periods of time which gradually became
longer as the exam day approached. This method reduced the stress
which I associated with studying because I had adequate time to absorb
information. When the exam day arrived, I was calm and had memorized
the material which was required to complete the exam.

THE EXAMINATION AND THE PROPER SETTING

Reduction of stress during exams is necessary for the dyslexic student to realize his full potential. For this reason, it is important for the exam to be structured properly and given in the proper setting on an untimed basis. The professor will usually offer to administer the exam along with the rest of the class or at a location which is secluded and quite. If the course causes the dyslexic student considerable difficulty, he should take the exam in a quiet, secluded location which is conducive to concentration.

EXAMINATIONS AND THE PROCESS OF INFORMATION ALTERATION

Inevitably, the dyslexic student will enroll in a course during college which he considers to be exceedingly difficult or boring. Exam material for this course will difficult for him to remember because it won't be interesting. Rather than feeling discouraged, he should alter the material in his mind so that it becomes interesting. For example: if a list of boring words must be memorized, he should think of words which sound similar to them but have some appeal. Once the boring words have been converted into interesting words, they may be used to form a short story. At this point, the boring words will be memorable because they have been given special significance; they are the basis for a story.

This procedure may also apply to other areas of study. A complex graph can be converted into a picture by using the lines to form objects. When graphs have been converted into pictures they are easier to remember and easier to draw because they represent simple pictures.

The dyslexic student has a superior capacity for creative thinking which he must use to cope with boring or perplexing work. The only disadvantage to this method of study is that it distorts information and stores it in the short-term memory. The created words and pictures have no relation to the subject matter which will not be learned using this method. I recommend this method of study only when conventional methods fail. It would be a shame for the dyslexic student to complete a course without learning the material, but it would be a tragedy if his GPA dropped to reflect this lack of knowledge.

THE UTILIZATION OF OFFICE HOURS TO OBTAIN EXAMINATION INFORMATION

When studying for an exam, students often have the option to discuss the subject with the professor or his teaching assistants during office hours. Although this time is allotted for students to receive guidance, the professor will state that he will not provide information for a test, but rather, that he will assist students to learn the information on their own. Although this explanation sounds good in theory, it is inaccurate in practice. Professors provide office hours to assist students in their understanding of the subject, therefore, a relationship exists wherein the professor provides information and the student receives. If the student can keep the professor talking about the subject, he will eventually reveal all pertinent information.

A student may succeed in receiving detailed information from a professor by formulating a basic set of questions which the professor must answer during a meeting. When the professor answers the first question, the student should restate this answer in a manner which suggests that he understands it only to a point. The professor will then provide a second answer which contains additional information to alleviate the lack of knowledge which has been displayed by his student. The student must then continue to his second question in order not to seem ignorant and then repeat the same process which he used for his first question. As the student proceeds to ask additional questions, he must relate these questions to information which has been provided in answers which the professor has given to previous questions. This pattern will cause the professor to divulge additional information which the student may use to improve his performance on class assignments which require him to demonstrate a good understanding of the course subject.

OVERCOMING READING PROBLEMS DURING STUDY

When studying, a common problem for dyslexics will be to simply read the material. This problem occurs because the dyslexic student thinks pictorially while the material he reads may be represented in a verbal/linear fashion. Even though the dyslexic may not understand a word when he reads it, he may understand the word if he hears it spoken in conversation. In order to overcome this problem, the dyslexic student must discover a means which will allow him to pictorially represent words which he does not understand. The solution will be for him to visualize a person speaking while he reads the material. This person should be someone who the dyslexic student has often seen speaking. This way, the dyslexic may pictorially create the image of a person who may speak to him through the text which he reads in order to improve comprehension.

METHODS TO OVERCOME MATHEMATICAL PROBLEMS

Another common problem which dyslexic students face is correctly solving simple mathematical problems. If an assignment requires addition or subtraction, the dyslexic student may incorrectly answer the question due to faulty calculations he makes as a result of his inability to pictorially represent the numbers in his mind. The solution to this dilemma is for him to pictorially visualize the mathematical problem in order to obtain the correct answer.

When calculating simple addition or subtraction, the dyslexic student should visualize a building (or similar physical structure) which contains one hundred rooms (or other units appropriate to the example). The units of this physical structure may be pictorially increased to comply with the requirements of larger mathematical problems (for example: one thousand units to solve mathematical problems which contain figures to be added or subtracted in the hundreds) The structure will appear pictorially in the dyslexic student's mind as indicated in figure 9.1.

If the dyslexic student must subtract eighty-three from one hundred, he may obtain an answer as indicated in figure 9.2.

If the dyslexic student must add twenty-three and forty-eight, the answer may be obtained as indicated in figure 9.3.

The number of rooms which the building contains will depend on the numbers which must be dealt with to find a solution to the problem. The example of a building is only one physical object of which the dyslexic student may conceive pictorially for this purpose. Another

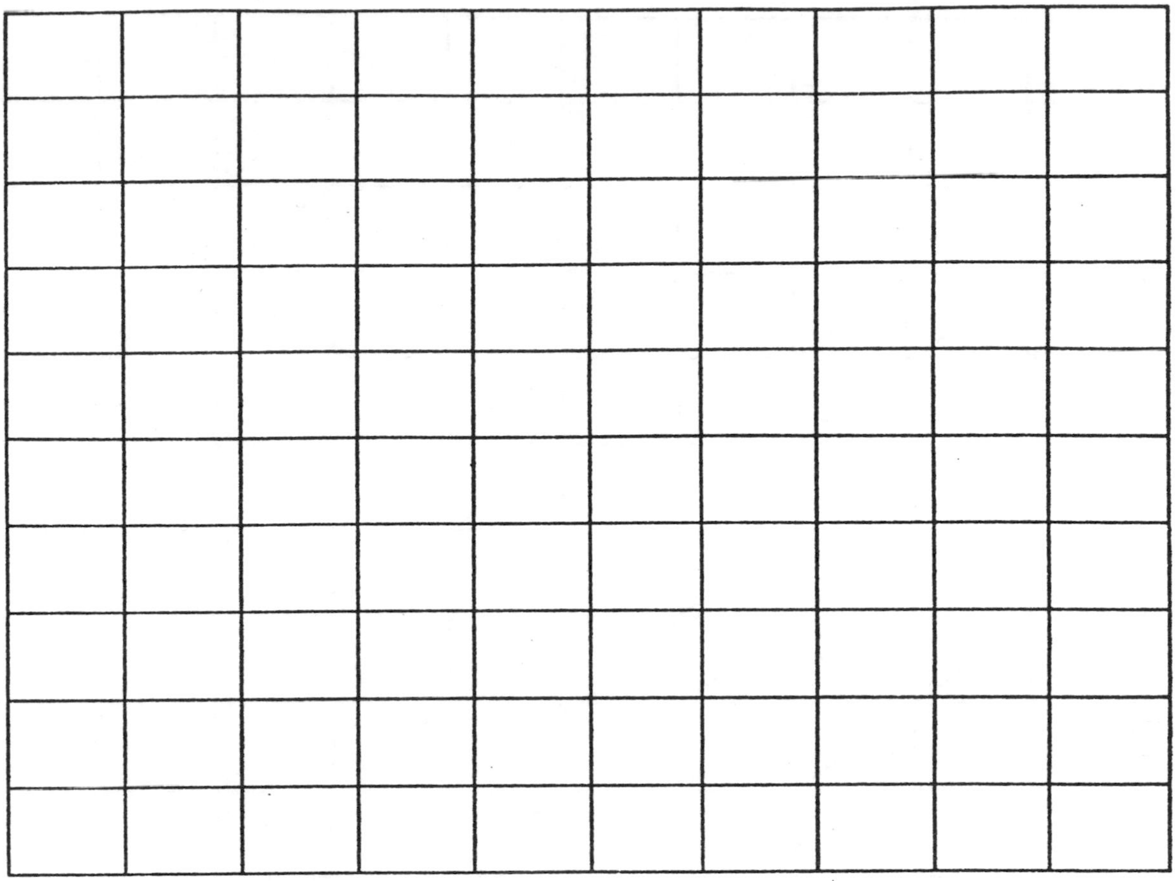

BASIS FOR PICTORIAL MATHEMATICAL PROBLEM-SOLVING

The above block of one hundred squares represents a building which contains one hundred rooms. This block may be used to pictorially represent numbers when solving mathematical problems.

Figure 9.1

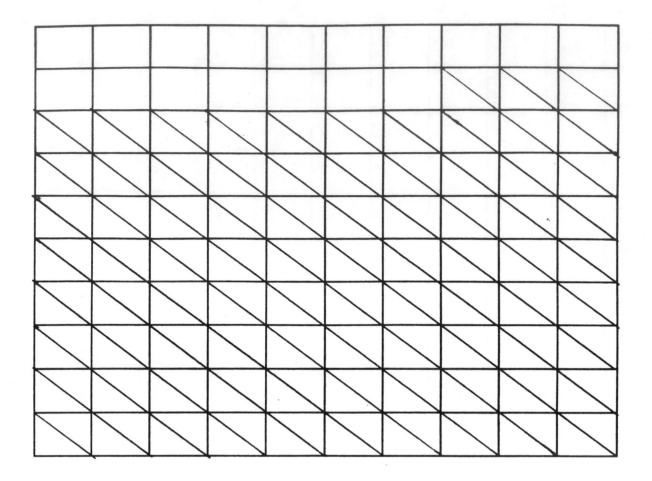

PICTORIAL SUBTRACTION EXAMPLE

The reader should imagine the above block of one hundred squares to be a one hundred room building in which all lights are turned on. Then, imagine that the lights in the bottom eighty-three rooms are suddenly turned off while the lights in the remaining seventeen rooms continue to shine. By following this simple procedure, the reader has pictorially solved the mathematical problem: one hundred minus eighty-three equals seventeen.

This procedure should be repeated every time the dyslexic student must quickly subtract numbers to solve mathematical problems. The number of rooms in the building may be increased to solve mathematical problems which involve higher numbers.

Figure 9.2

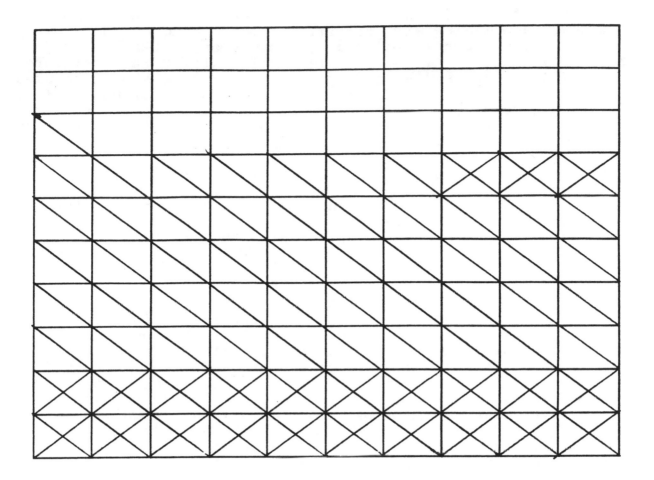

PICTORIAL ADDITION EXAMPLE

The reader should imagine the above block of one hundred squares to be
a building in which all lights are turned off. Then, imagine that the
bottom twenty lights are turned on immediately followed by the forty
lights which comprise the third, fourth, fifth, and sixth floors. At
this point, the lights of the bottom six floors are turned on. Now,
imagine that three of the lights on the seventh floor are turned on,
immediately followed by the next eight. At this point, seventy-one
lights are turned on while twenty-nine lights are turned off. The
reader has just pictorially solved the mathematical problem:
twenty-three plus forty-eight equals seventy-one.

Figure 9.3

object may suffice when numbers become larger than one hundred because the image of a building will be limited to one hundred rooms.

When the above mentioned procedure has been mastered, it should be used everyday to overcome mathematical difficulties in the future. When goods are purchased at a store, this procedure should be used to add individual sums and determine the change that will be received from a larger banknote. If this procedure is used regularly, the dyslexic student should be able to add and subtract faster than he ever believed was possible.

LEARNING TO "READ" AN EXAM

In addition to good study techniques, it will be important for the dyslexic student to learn how to "read" an exam. Professors often divulge information in the manner in which they ask exam questions. Reading an exam is a technique whereby a student answers an exam question using information which has been divulged in other exam questions. For example, an exam question asks "Which of the following is not a form of government? A) democratic B) socialist C) fascist D) Buddhist". If the student chooses "D", he may correctly answer 75% of another exam question in which he must identify four types of government. Reading an exam allows the dyslexic student to compensate for information that has been forgotten or overlooked when studying. It may help to view the exam as a jigsaw puzzle which offers several pieces of information which must fit together in order to obtain an answer to the question. This technique compliments studying, but it may never be used as a substitute because the answers which are given to exam questions must be correct if the dyslexic student is to use this information to answer other questions.

STRESS REDUCTION AND THE EXAMINATION

During an exam, a point may be reached where the dyslexic student is uncertain or unaware of the answer to an exam question. The natural response to this situation will be to experience a fear of failure which will cause stress. This emotional response will cause the dyslexic student to do poorly on the exam because it will stifle his mind's ability to subconsciously solve the problem and will prevent him from correctly answering other questions for which he already possesses the correct knowledge.

In order to overcome stress when encountering an exam question for which no answer is apparent, the dyslexic student should close his eyes and forget that he is taking an exam. He should then remember an activity in which he excels and recall his emotional response when he succeeds at this activity. This memory will cause the dyslexic student to acquire a heightened state of conscious awareness. While focusing all attention on the activity in which the dyslexic excels, he must then open his eyes and view the exam question with the thought that he already has the answer in his mind. At this point, his subconscious mind will provide an answer to the exam question. He may then complete the exam without suffering the negative results which are associated with stress.

In order to illustrate the extent to which this technique works, I will provide an example from my past. During my senior year in high school, I registered to take the SAT timed because I was unaware that I was entitled to receive accommodations. I knew that I would graduate in the top ten percent of my high school class, so I experienced no stress during the exam because the results would not be considered by college admissions officers.

I was required to answer questions involving abstract mathematics and English on the SAT. I had previously done well in high school English classes, so I strove to make a grade in the English section of the test which would reflect this knowledge. As a result of my concentration, I was unable to complete all English questions within the allotted time. When I encountered the abstract mathematics section of the test, I could not understand the questions because I had only completed introductory algebra during high school. I answered the mathematical questions by trying to "guess" the correct answer from the options given. I viewed this exercise as a game because I could not understand the abstract mathematical questions and I was curious to know how many I could answer based on a chance theory. In order to do this, I would look at an abstract mathematical question and choose the answer which seemed to be most appealing.

When the test was completed, I had answered all abstract mathematical questions because I had taken no time to calculate the answers. I had managed to answer only a portion of the English questions because I had given each one careful consideration. I was shocked when I received the results of the test. I had obtained a score of 410 for the abstract mathematical questions out of a possible 800, and I had obtained a score of 400 for the English questions out of a possible 800. Because I had experienced no stress when I answered the abstract mathematical questions, I instructed my subconscious mind to choose the correct answers from the available options. As a result, my subconscious mind correctly solved more than fifty percent of the abstract mathematical questions, the processes for which my conscious mind could not even comprehend! The same technique can work for any subject if the dyslexic student learns how to master the technique of subconscious problem-solving.

THE DYSLEXIC STUDENT AND THE WRITTEN ASSIGNMENT

The dyslexic student will also be required to complete written assignments such as term papers and essay exams. As is the case with all exams, written assignments may also be changed or substituted if this manner of testing conflicts with dyslexia. Written assignments are more complicated than most exams because they require the student to understand and apply the material which has been studied in class, rather than simply memorize it. It is impossible to guess on written assignments because the grade is based on the student's ability to creatively demonstrate his knowledge of the course material.

A written assignment has two advantages over other forms of exams: more time is available to prepare for a written assignment and a rough draft of the written assignment may usually be submitted to the professor for review. This review allows the student to correct mistakes before submitting the final draft. Written assignments should be prepared by choosing a topic when the instruction sheet is received from the professor which explains his requirements. The dyslexic student should begin to prepare the rough draft immediately after he receives the instruction sheet. The dyslexic student may decide to change the topic based on problems which he encounters in the beginning. If the decision is made to change topics, the dyslexic student will have plenty of time to write another assignment because he will be ahead of schedule. When the rough draft is completed, it should be submitted to the professor for evaluation in order to have ample time to make corrections. If the professor's evaluation is unclear, it should be discussed with him to be certain what corrections must be made and for what reason. Once the professor's evaluation of the rough draft is clear, the dyslexic student will be ready to prepare his final draft.

A written assignment should never be submitted earlier than those of the other students in the class because the professor will have more time to find fault with it. Instead, written assignments should be held and submitted at the deadline. The professor will have the other written assignments to grade so he will be unlikely to discover all mistakes in the dyslexic student's written assignment due to time constraints. For this reason, it is better to enroll in large, rather than small, classes when both require written assignments. The size of the class will not affect the professor's availability to the dyslexic student because he is a special student who is entitled to special attention. When the graded written assignment is received, the dyslexic student may find that he has been given a better grade than he feels he deserves. However, if the grade appears to be too low, it should be discussed with the professor in an attempt to convince him that it should be risen. The dyslexic student must always remember that the professor serves his students, therefore, students should never risk their GPA to accommodate his schedule by submitting written assignments before the deadline.

Problems may arise during essay exams because of limited time which is available to prepare answers and because the professor must read the dyslexic student's handwriting. When faced with an impending essay exam, the dyslexic student should contact the professor and ask what types of questions will be asked on the exam and request a sheet of sample questions from which to study. This sheet and the professor's comments will help to clarify what information he considers to be most important. The professor must be informed that handwriting and spelling may be poor due to dyslexia so that he will not deduct points in these areas. The dyslexic student should offer to read his essays to the professor after the exam if they appear unclear to him. This action will show the professor that the dyslexic student is cooperative and concerned about course work.

Chapter Ten
WHEN CONFLICT ARISES

During college years, the dyslexic student may encounter conflict with professors or college administrators due to accommodations which must be made to accurately assess his knowledge of course work. In most cases, conflict is handled on an administrative level through mutual agreement between the dyslexic student and the college. Although no conflict is pleasant, the dyslexic student may consider himself fortunate because he currently enjoys more legal protection than at any time before. This legal protection exists due to the passage of the Americans With Disabilities Act which specifically defines the college's responsibility to accommodate dyslexic students.

RECOMMENDATIONS FOR CONFLICT RESOLUTION

Only five years ago, American colleges were free to establish exclusion policies against dyslexic applicants and require dyslexic students to complete college courses without providing accommodations because the laws which existed at that time to protect dyslexics had been weakened and were easy to evade. It was also a common practice for colleges to require dyslexic students to complete courses which focused on subjects which they couldn't comprehend, given the verbal/linear methods of instruction which were provided. Without adequate methods of instruction, dyslexic students were forced to leave college after their grades had fallen below acceptable levels. Fortunately, this situation no longer exists, but caution is still warranted when dealing with professors and administrators during conflicts.

In view of new legislation which protects dyslexic American citizens, the reader might never encounter a situation in college in which he would benefit from the information contained in this chapter, however, I would be negligent in my responsibility to the reader if I were to assume that conflict will never arise in college as a result of new legislation. For this reason, I provide the following recommendations for the dyslexic student to deal with conflict which I hope never comes to pass during the college years.

First, when the dyslexic student contacts his college to resolve a conflict, he should obtain all agreements in writing from administrators in order to have proof that the agreement exists. Administrators often change jobs and those who remain may not correctly recall the details of the agreement which has been reached.

Second, always request that the administrators provide an estimation of how long it will take to resolve the conflict, even if the administrators only act as arbitrators to resolve an academic conflict with a professor. A common practice which was used by administrators during my college years was to delay action as long as possible when I requested intervention to resolve a conflict, and then fail to act when I appealed to a higher authority because I had waited too long to appeal. Once administrators have committed themselves to a time limit, they must be held to it.

Third, when conflict arises, the disabled students' association must be notified along with a request for their assistance to resolve the conflict. Once they have agreed to provide assistance, the dyslexic student should find out exactly what they will do and how long it will take. Then, the Rehab office (or another organization for the disabled if desirable) must be contacted in order for them to refer the matter to someone in their legal department. This person must be given a full explanation of the conflict along with a report of the action which has been taken and who in the administration has been contacted. If the disabled students' association fails to resolve the conflict, they must be contacted by the legal advocate directly to obtain an explanation. This way, the disabled students' association may work in cooperation with a person who has authority and expertise in the law. If the conflict remains unresolved, the administration may be blamed for having failed to act when appeals are made to higher authorities for intervention to resolve the conflict.

Finally, the dyslexic student has access to one resource which may prove invaluable when dealing with conflict: the media. Colleges spend considerable time and money to promote positive images of themselves in order to attract new students. Conflict will usually be resolved quickly if the dyslexic student is willing to use the media to broadcast his case to the American people. This publicity will place the college's public image in jeopardy and also risk their state and federal funds which they receive on the condition that they comply with the law. Failure to comply with the law may result in the State and Federal Governments withholding these funds.

THE TECHNIQUE OF IMAGE CONVEYANCE

When attempting to resolve conflict with a college, the dyslexic student must convey the correct image of himself in order to prevail. The mutual perceptions which exist between the dyslexic student and the administration depend upon the images which each hold of the other. For this reason, it will be beneficial for the dyslexic student to convey an image to the administration which will inhibit their ability to anticipate the actions which he will take to resolve the conflict.

The key to successfully resolving conflict with a college administration, or any bureaucratic organization, is to understand the technique of image conveyance. This technique is based on the assumption that the level of opposition which a person provides in a conflict will be determined by the intelligence which he perceives in his opponent. If a person can control his opponent's perception of his intelligence, then he can minimize, and often predict, the steps which his opponent will take against him and take action beforehand to counter these moves. In order to better explain this technique, I will focus on the three categories of people who challenge authority.

In the first category is the person who reacts to opposition by conveying an image of himself which suggests that he is more intelligent than is the case. This person realizes that his opponent possesses superior intelligence and attempts to defeat his opponent by posing a challenge to his intelligence. In this case, the opponent simply creates a situation which requires this person to demonstrate the extent of his intelligence. When this person is unable to compete on his opponent's intellectual level, it becomes apparent that he possesses inferior intelligence. He is defeated when this lack of knowledge destroys his credibility in the eyes of the arbitrator who favors his opponent who has demonstrated superior intelligence.

In the second category is the person who reacts to opposition by conveying an image of himself which suggests that he is neither more nor less intelligent than is the case. This person has a better chance of success than the person of the first category because he approaches the conflict without pretenses. He presents his case against that of his opponent and leaves the resolution of the conflict to the decision of the arbitrator. The problem which he faces is that his opponent possesses greater knowledge which will likely diminish his chance to obtain an acceptable resolution.

In the third category is the person who reacts to opposition by conveying an image of himself which suggests that he is less intelligent than is the case. This person has the best chance for success because his opponent will be unable to correctly anticipate the level of opposition which will be required to defeat this person. By conveying an image of himself as a person of limited intelligence, the person of the third category benefits in two ways: First, he reinforces his opponent's self-image of superiority. Second, he controls the level of opposition which he will receive by giving his opponent a false sense of security. An opponent will devise a strategy to combat conflict based upon the level of opposition which he expects to receive. If he perceives the person of the third category to be of limited intelligence, he will formulate his strategy with this thought in mind. He will also anticipate a resolution to the conflict which supports his position due to the fact that this person's perceived lack of intelligence has reinforced his feelings of superiority.

When both cases are presented before the arbitrator, the person of the third category who conveyed an image of himself as being of limited intelligence will present his case in a manner which reflects his full knowledge and capability. This sophisticated presentation will come as a surprise to his opponent who had believed him to be a person of limited intelligence. In this case, it will be the opponent who appears to be of limited intelligence because he will present a case which has been prepared to combat a person of limited intelligence. In order to fully benefit from this situation, the person of the third category must call attention to the fact that his opponent is unorganized and seemingly unprepared to address the points of discussion. The opponent will likely become angry when he realizes that he has underestimated the person of the third category, at which time he may appear to be highly emotional before the arbitrator while the person of the third category presents his case calmly and professionally.

APPROACHES TO MAXIMIZE THE EFFECTIVENESS OF IMAGE CONVEYANCE

In order to approach conflict as a person of the third category, the dyslexic student must do the following: First, at the point when it becomes obvious that the professor or administrator will be unwilling to negotiate a resolution to the conflict, and that outside arbitration will be required, he should not reveal his plans to seek arbitration. This knowledge will give his opponent time to contact his allies within the administration to block the dyslexic student's efforts.

Second, the dyslexic student should review American law and school policy regarding his particular case in order to formulate a success strategy to defeat his opponent. If he can show that favorable action has been taken in similar cases, he may argue that these cases have set precedents which should be applied to the resolution of his conflict.

Third, when a strategy has been formulated to defeat his opponent, the dyslexic student must contact people who he suspects are loyal to his opponent and mention to them that he wishes to seek arbitration to resolve the conflict. It will be best if these people have never met him because they will have no past impressions regarding his level of intelligence.

Fourth, while speaking with these people, the dyslexic student should ask questions which suggest that he lacks basic knowledge of college policy and procedures in order for them to believe that he is of limited intelligence. These people may tell his opponent about the meeting and convey the message to his opponent that he is of limited intelligence because he asked questions which revealed a significant lack of knowledge.

Fifth, immediately after speaking with the opponent's associates, the dyslexic student should contact someone within the college administration whom he considers to be fair. This person must be informed of the conflict along with a request for arbitration. He should also be someone who already believes the dyslexic student to be intelligent. This image will allow the dyslexic student to easily portray himself during arbitration as an intelligent person who wishes to resolve conflict through administrative channels.

Sixth, once a meeting time and an arbitrator have been arranged, the dyslexic student should contact his opponent and notify him that an appeal has been made to a higher authority. The opponent should be provided only the information which he is required to know, such as the time and location of the meeting. The dyslexic student should spend the time which remains before the meeting preparing his arguments and attempting to find inconsistencies in the school's policies which may work to his advantage.

CONFLICT RESOLUTION THROUGH THE CONTRADICTION OF BELIEF SYSTEMS

When conflict is encountered in college, it will be beneficial if arguments are presented in relation to the beliefs which are held by the person with whom the dyslexic student is engaged in conflict, or the arbitrator if the conflict may not be resolved through direct dialogue with this person. A person will justify his actions in accordance with the system of beliefs which he holds. If a person is shown that his actions are in conflict with his system of beliefs, then he will likely change his actions to conform to these beliefs.

I met a young woman named Sveta in Dallas last year who had immigrated from Ukraine two years earlier. Although English was her second language, she had mastered it well enough to earn a 3.89 GPA in community college. As she completed her sophomore year, she was in the process of choosing a university where she would transfer in order to complete her final two years of college. Due to her exceptional GPA, she had been accepted to a number of reputable colleges, however, she wished to remain in Dallas and live with her family while attending a local university. In order to defer college expenses, she applied to receive financial assistance from a number of scholarships which had been established to benefit college students who had achieved her level of academic success.

One evening, Sveta told me that she faced an academic crisis. It seems that the college financial aid office had incorrectly informed her that the deadline for submitting scholarship applications was May 3, when in fact the correct deadline was March 3. The date at the time of our conversation was March 9. Her family was most distressed because she had missed the deadline due to misinformation which she had received from the financial aid office. In an attempt to resolve the conflict, Sveta made three telephone calls to the director of the financial aid office to explain the misunderstanding, yet the director claimed that Sveta was at fault and there was nothing he could do to correct the situation.

Sveta believed that she had lost thousands of dollars due to an error which had been made by a clerk in the financial aid office. Without the additional money, she would have been unable to graduate in a two-year period due to the fact that she would have to maintain full-time employment while attending college in order to pay the additional expenses.

Upon hearing of this situation, I realized that Sveta's failure to prevail in this conflict was the result of her inability to formulate an effective success strategy. After receiving all details from Sveta, we both visited the university to discuss the conflict with the university administration. I did not talk to the director of the financial aid office because he had made his position on the matter perfectly clear during his three telephone conversations with Sveta. Instead, I consulted the dean of admissions to explain the conflict and obtain his recommendations for potential resolutions. He initially suggested that I contact the director of the financial aid office. I explained the lack of cooperation which Sveta had received from this man and I asked the dean for names of appropriate members of administration who could overrule the director of the financial aid office in this matter. He suggested that I speak to the university vice-president and provost, so I proceeded to the administration building where I met the university vice-president and explained the conflict.

At first, the vice-president supported the position which had been taken by the director of the financial aid office, however, I succeeded in presenting my case in such a manner that opposition would conflict with the system of beliefs which he held regarding the function of the education system and his role within it.

I began by explaining to him that the conflict had occurred due to an administrative error which had been made on the part of a clerk in the financial aid office. As I expected, he refuted my claim by stating that Sveta had misunderstood the clerk. I countered by stating that Sveta had mastered English as a second language so well that she had earned a 3.89 GPA in college, therefore, it would have been unlikely that she had misunderstood the information which had been given regarding submission deadlines. I then added that it was virtually impossible for her to misunderstand the correct deadline for filing scholarship applications because her ability to attend the university would depend upon her receiving financial assistance.

The vice-president considered my arguments for a couple of seconds and retorted that the clerks in the financial aid office were very well trained and would not provide incorrect information regarding deadlines. I then asked him if applicants for financial assistance had ever reported that they had received incorrect information from the financial aid office regarding deadlines. He admitted that such cases had occurred, but he hastened to add that the university had determined that the applicants were at fault in these cases and had supported the position held by the financial aid office. I then asked the vice-president if he believed that it was possible that some of these students had received incorrect information from the financial aid office. He conceded that it was possible, however, he stated that he personally believed that the majority of these applicants had failed to submit application due to their own failings. I responded by asking him if he believed that applicants should be denied financial assistance if they comply with incorrect instructions which they have received from officials within the financial aid office.

He considered my question for several seconds and then responded that students definitely should not be held responsible for mistakes which have been made by the financial aid office, however, he concluded that the university could not make exceptions for one applicant because this action would set a precedent which would obligate the university to take similar action in future cases. I responded by stating that a university exists to meet the needs of its students and explained the ordeals which Sveta had endured in order to achieve the high GPA which had qualified her to attend his university. The vice-president told me that he sympathized with Sveta's problem, but added that he knew no way in which the conflict could be resolved through administrative intervention. I responded by stating that Sveta's conflict was a case in which the administration's procedures conflicted with the very purpose of the university. Then, in a tone of voice which appealed to reason, I stated that Sveta, after having worked so hard to be eligible to attend his university, was now being punished because she had followed instructions which she had received from university representatives.

The vice-president pondered my last statement for fifteen seconds, could think of no retort, and excused himself while he went into his office and called the director of the financial aid office to discuss a resolution to Sveta's conflict. The call lasted for several minutes and it was obvious from excerpts I overheard that the director of the financial aid office did not approve of administrative action which would overrule his decision to deny Sveta the right to submit financial aid applications. The vice-president soon returned and informed us that he had spoken with the director of the financial aid office who had agreed to allow her to submit her financial aid applications, even though the deadline had passed. Sveta and I then went to the financial aid office where we received application forms from the director for Sveta to receive financial assistance.

When the application forms had been completed, Sveta presented them to the secretary and I requested that the director personally write a letter for Sveta which stated that her application had been submitted and accepted beyond the deadline with his approval. The secretary returned several minutes later with signed copies of the application forms on which the director had written that they had been submitted beyond the deadline with his approval. I then proceeded to contact the vice-president and the secretary of the university provost who had agreed to oversee the case and thanked them for the assistance they had provided.

ANALYSIS OF A SUCCESSFUL APPROACH

In this situation, Sveta had been unable to formulate an effective success strategy because she was unaware of the methods required to present her argument in relation to the belief system held by the university vice-president. When we met the vice-president, he conveyed the arguments which were customary to deal with applicants who request extensions for submitting applications. I prevailed in this conflict because I was able to show the vice-president that these arguments conflicted with his beliefs regarding the function of a university, the rights of applicants, and his function as the university vice-president. I also prevailed because I approached the meeting as a person who was attempting to correct an administrative error rather than a person who was attempting to exact special treatment which conflicted with administrative procedures.

Every time the vice-president suggested that Sveta was at fault, I suggested that the university was at fault and proceeded with the objective of finding an administrative solution to this error. The vice-president's opposition ended when he was unable to provide additional arguments to refute my position. He then contacted another member of the university administration in support of the same position which he had only minutes earlier attempted to refute. At that point, Sveta's administrative solution had been found.

During this conflict, I viewed my opponent to be the director of the financial aid office who had so rudely refused to consider Sveta's reasons for failing to submit her applications before the deadline. I defeated this man because I manipulated the same university system of rules and regulations which he had used to prevent Sveta from receiving financial assistance. I requested the written confirmation of her financial aid application submission as proof of his acceptance and also as tangible evidence that he had conceded defeat in this conflict to a man who he had never met before and will likely never meet again.

THREE CHALLENGES TO THE COMPLETION OF A SUCCESSFUL APPROACH

I encountered many situations at The University of Texas at Austin which required me to demonstrate to administrators that their positions in various matters conflicted with their beliefs. This success strategy for conflict resolution is extremely effective, however, it also presents three challenges to the dyslexic student.

First, the dyslexic student must achieve a heightened state of conscious awareness in order to adequately combat arguments presented by the administrator. If these arguments are not quickly refuted, the dyslexic student will appear to be slow and uncertain of his position. Every argument which the administrator presents must be refuted with the same conviction in order for the dyslexic student to be truly effective. The dyslexic student must use his natural ability to view the world through the administrator's eyes in order to adequately refute his arguments. If the dyslexic student cannot correctly understand the way in which the administrator thinks, it will be difficult to refute his position.

Second, the dyslexic student must be convinced that his position is correct. The administrator will prevail if he convinces the dyslexic student that the administration's position is correct. For this reason, it will be necessary for the dyslexic student to convince himself that he has defeated the administrator before the meeting begins. If the subconscious mind believes that victory has been obtained, it will provide the dyslexic student arguments which he may use to refute the administrator's position. If the dyslexic student is concerned about the outcome of the meeting, his subconscious mind will not function to its full potential due to negative influences and failure will be the likely result.

Third, the dyslexic student must present his case in a manner which does not involve the excessive use of words. A case which is presented using few words will be more effective because it illustrates the dyslexic student's ability to organize his thoughts in a concise manner. It also causes the listener to carefully evaluate the information provided because he has more time to analyze each of the dyslexic student's points. In my previous example, I overcame objections made by the university vice-president through the use of short statements and by asking simple questions which caused him to evaluate Sveta's conflict in relation to his own beliefs and self-image. The conflict was resolved, not as a result of my words, but rather, as a result of the conclusions which my words caused him to draw in his own mind during the periods when he paused.

Overcoming administrative opposition through the presentation of arguments conveyed through the use of few words will be a most effective tactic for the dyslexic student to use when formulating success strategies. Arguments will be more convincing if the listener agrees with the dyslexic student's points through his own reasoning processes, rather than through attempts to persuade him by presenting all information which pertains to the case. Just as a joke is humorous because the listener realizes the underlying message in his own mind, so too may an argument be convincing if the listener draws the conclusion that a position is correct through his own process of reasoning. On the other hand, an argument which is conveyed through the excessive use of words will be least effective because the listener will believe that the speaker is trying to obtain his approval by inundating him with more information than his mind can effectively comprehend.

When attempting to resolve conflict before an arbitrator, the dyslexic student must always remain calm and present his arguments effectively. He must never become angry. The opponent may become angry if he wishes; this behavior will only strengthen the argument that the dyslexic student is being treated unfairly. In some instances, the college will request that the dyslexic student sign an agreement when a conflict is resolved. The legal advocate must always read any agreement which the college wishes the dyslexic student to sign. The document may appear normal to the dyslexic student, however, documents can be deceiving and he may agree to something by signing that will be harmful in the future.

In conclusion, I would like to point out that there always exist exceptions to college policies when these policies inhibit a dyslexic student's learning processes. Reluctance to provide accommodations is more a reflection of attitudes held by individual professors and administrators than it is of the flexibility of the college to adapt its procedures to benefit the dyslexic student.

At the beginning of this chapter, I conveyed my hope that academic conflicts will never arise in which the information contained within this chapter would be useful. Although the rights of dyslexics to receive accommodations in college have recently been fortified, such conflicts may arise for unpredictable reasons. In the event that the reader is unable to benefit in college from the information provided in this chapter, I am certain that conflicts will arise at some point which will offer the opportunity to utilize this information.

Chapter Eleven
LIFE AFTER COLLEGE

One day, barring unforeseen catastrophe, the dyslexic student will graduate from college. This ceremony will not only celebrate his ability to complete required courses, it will also demonstrate his ability to prevail within a bureaucratic institution. When he walks onto the stage to receive his diploma, he will be overcome by a feeling of triumph. Although pride will certainly be justified, his situation will not have improved from the day he enrolled in college unless he formulates a success strategy which will allow him to achieve his goals. A graduating senior has four basic options with regard to the future: 1) corporate employment 2) government employment 3) entrepreneurship 4) graduate school.

THE DYSLEXIC GRADUATE AND CORPORATE EMPLOYMENT

Corporate employment is the most alluring option to most dyslexic graduates because it provides the opportunity for them to convert their abilities into financial rewards. Dyslexic graduates possess advantages over other applicants because they were required to work hard to overcome obstacles to the comprehension of college course work, they have overcome administrative conflicts, and they have mastered the art of bureaucracy manipulation. In a perfect world, dyslexic graduates would be the most sought after applicants for corporate employment. Unfortunately, we do not live in a perfect world and business recruiters may hold stereotypes which will limit the dyslexic graduate's ability to obtain corporate employment.

A recruiter selects applicants whom he feels will provide the greatest benefit for the company he represents. The dyslexic graduate is considered to be disabled and will likely require special accommodations in the event that he receives employment. Recruiters seldom realize the advantages of hiring dyslexic graduates, and as a result, may view the dyslexic as a person who has a problem. Although the Americans With Disabilities Act protects dyslexics from job discrimination, it is difficult for the dyslexic applicant to know if he has been rejected on the basis of his dyslexia or because other applicants have been chosen due to superior qualifications.

Another technique which a recruiter may use to avoid hiring dyslexic applicants is to prolong the interviewing process so long that the dyslexic applicant either loses interest or finds another job. Little recourse may be available in this instance because it is impossible to prove that he is the victim of discrimination rather than bureaucracy. In this regard, it may be said that some companies have an affirmative inaction policy: definitely doing nothing.

RESOURCES TO ACHIEVE CORPORATE EMPLOYMENT

It will not be beneficial for the dyslexic student to conduct a job search without assistance. Instead, he should contact organizations that exist to help dyslexics and explain his qualifications, degree, and the type of employment which he hopes to obtain. These organizations may have links with people in the business community who realize the creative potential of dyslexics and might be interested to provide a job interview. The dyslexic student must be wary of organizations that exist to assist college graduates obtain employment. The two organizations most frequently used by recent graduates are the college placement office and employment agencies.

The college placement office exists to assist in the graduate's search for employment, however, they are seldom able to provide employment which meets their goals because the number of college graduates seeking employment far outweighs the number of companies which seek employees. As a result, the college placement office must work hard to locate companies that are willing to hire graduates. Companies realize that they may choose from many qualified applicants, so they often offer less than the average salary for positions which they wish to fill. An applicant will inevitably accept the company's job offer and the director of the college placement office will seldom interfere because he needs the company's support far more than the company needs applicants which are provided by the placement office.

If the dyslexic student chooses to conduct a job search with the assistance of a college placement office, he should contact the competitors of any company with which he wishes to interview with the assistance of the placement office and make an inquiry regarding the salary which these companies offer applicants for the same position. If the competitors offer a higher salary, he should apply for employment with these companies instead of the companies to which he would apply with the assistance of the placement office.

A second organization frequently used by college graduates is the employment agency. Beware of the employment agency that charges fees to applicants rather than their client companies. Employment agencies provide applicants as a service to client companies, so the applicant should never pay fees to the employment agency for services which benefit client companies. For this reason, it is important for applicants to thoroughly read the content of any contracts provided by the employment agency. Employment agencies which charge fees to client companies may avoid conflicts of interest between the needs of applicants and client companies, however, the applicant may still experience conflict because the employment agency serves the client company's interests as well as those of the applicant.

Employment agencies may be divided into two separate categories: executive search agencies and temporary employment agencies. Executive search agencies offer positions to applicants who satisfy the strict requirements of client companies which search for management personnel. These companies are usually well established in their markets and often appear on the Fortune 500 list of leading companies in America. Applicants who are accepted by executive search agencies must demonstrate leadership abilities and earned high GPAs while in college.

The executive search agency provides the most qualified college graduates the opportunity to obtain management positions immediately after graduation rather than having to accept lesser positions from which to advance into management positions. The executive search agency is a good option for the dyslexic graduate who has achieved a high degree of success in college because the competition to obtain management positions is reduced due to strict employment requirements for the positions they offer. The dyslexic graduate benefits from the executive search agency because he receives more personal attention from agency personnel. The reputation of the executive search agency depends upon its ability to place applicants in positions where they are compatible with employers.

The temporary employment agency is most commonly used by the dyslexic college graduate as a means to obtain employment during the period when he conducts his search for permanent employment. The temporary employment agency serves the needs of the business community by providing employees to fill positions which involve clerical work, sales, trades, and manual labor. The client company pays the temporary employment agency a commission for locating and screening applicants to fill the various positions which they offer. The applicant rarely pays the temporary employment agency because the agency exists to provide acceptable applicants for their client companies. The applicant benefits from the temporary employment agency because the agency saves him from having to conduct a job search which could consume extensive time and energy.

The temporary employment business is currently one of the three fastest-growing industries in America due to changes which have taken place in American business philosophy. Whereas ten years ago an applicant might have believed that his employment with one company would last for decades if he were productive, the current job market is in a constant state of flux due to corporate America's need to reduce operating expenses in order to compete on the international market. Temporary agencies provide applicants for positions which would have been offered with a guarantee of job security only a decade ago. Today, American companies reduce employment expenses by hiring temporary workers who are provided no job security or benefits. Benefits are provided only when these temporary employees have demonstrated their ability to perform in accordance with the company's expectations.

THE DYSLEXIC GRADUATE AND THE MULTILEVEL MARKETING COMPANY

The dyslexic college graduate who conducts an independent job search must beware of companies which attempt to lure applicants by offering deceptive business opportunities. These companies often operate under a multilevel marketing structure in which the applicant works as an independent business person to sell products or services offered by the company. In many cases, applicants to these companies are required to purchase company handbooks or product samples which they are expected to show potential customers. Applicants who are accepted for these positions are paid a commission based on the amount of products which they sell and are encouraged to recruit other people to sell the same products in order to receive a commission.

The multilevel marketing industry thrives on applicants who have failed in their attempts to obtain suitable employment. They offer group interviews in which applicants are indoctrinated into the philosophy of the company and informed about the products which the company offers. The multilevel marketing company uses sophisticated persuasion techniques to convince applicants to sell their products while the management is aware that the vast majority of applicants are unsuitable for the position and will fail as a result.

I recently attended a group interview for a multilevel marketing company in order to examine the techniques which the company used to persuade applicants to join. The following description will provide a good example of the multilevel marketing approach:

The group interview began at 7:00 PM in an office building which was located in an upper middle-class suburb of Dallas. Approximately fifty applicants attended the interview which was conducted by the vice-president of the company who wore an expensive suit and spoke with an air of confidence which bordered on condescension. He began by providing a brief history of his company and explained that its founders had become multimillionaires through the use of a multilevel marketing scheme to sell products to the public which they had purchased directly from producers. The vice-president made several points about his company which he immediately followed with jokes and humorous statements to which company representatives seated in the audience responded by laughing. In the beginning, the audience was somewhat reserved regarding the company and its products, however, the association of humor with every point made by the speaker caused the audience to associate positive feelings with his points. The atmosphere in the room evolved from reservation in the beginning of the lecture to elation by the time the group interview had ended.

The function performed by the vice-president was to eliminate the beliefs which the audience held regarding their lack of abilities and to exploit feelings of inadequacy which had resulted from their failure to obtain suitable employment. In order to accomplish this task, the speaker identified with the audience by claiming that his company had been founded by people who were in similar situations which the members of the audience faced at the time. He proceeded to give examples of famous companies which had been founded by people in similar circumstances in order to lend credence to the information which he had provided regarding his own company.

When speaking about the possibility of working with his company, the vice-president would constantly make references to expensive cars and large homes while, at the same time, speaking of the insecurity of the American job market and the unlikelihood that Social Security would survive long enough for the members of the audience to collect benefits. This contrast created a feeling of acceptance among the members of the audience toward his company while it enhanced their fears of failing to find stable employment with companies that offered high wages and benefits.

Throughout the group interview, the vice-president provided examples of reputable institutions which allegedly had expressed support for his company. He also made frequent statements that his company's products were in such demand by the public that little persuasion would be required on the part of applicants to sell the products. The vice-president concluded his speech by revealing a roll of hundred-dollar bills in an attempt to locate a one-dollar bill on the back of which he hoped to demonstrate that even the founding fathers of the United States had supported pyramid schemes.

The group interview had been a success, judging from the number of applicants who enthusiastically expressed their desire to join the company. They had been persuaded by the vice-president's techniques, however, they failed to identify the inaccuracy of his arguments.

First, an applicant's income depended upon his ability to continually contact people who would purchase products. For this reason, the applicant could conceivably encounter a situation in which the commission he would receive from the sale of products would be less than the expenses of time and travel which he would incur to market the products to potential customers. If an applicant was without a large circle of friends and business contacts, he would be required to contact strangers in hopes that they would be receptive to his sales attempts.

Second, the examples of successful entrepreneurs which the vice-president provided had become wealthy only because they invested in new companies. The vice-president could not justify the comparison he made between his company and those which he used as examples because his company was an industry leader at the time of the group interview. By the time an applicant interviews with the multilevel marketing company, it is usually large enough to employ several thousand sales representatives with whom the new applicant must compete in order to survive in the market.

Third, the risk which applicants would assume was underemphasized while the potential reward offered by the company was overemphasized. As a result, the applicant was given inaccurate information on which to base his decision, thus assuming a much greater risk than he was willing or able to withstand.

The persuasion techniques used by multilevel marketing companies are similar to the techniques which have historically been used by communist governments to control the thoughts of their people because the conclusion to which these companies lead their applicants neither reflects reality nor is in the interest of the applicants themselves. These techniques are most harmful to the applicants because they give them a false sense of security which will ultimately be shattered when they are unable to sell sufficient quantities of the product to pay their living expenses. In this case, the applicants' self-esteem is severely damaged because they believe that they have failed to achieve a task which had been described to them as being simple and requiring little effort. The multilevel marketing company, on the other hand, receives money for any written material or products which the applicants purchase, in addition to the proceeds from any sales they make. For this income, the multilevel marketing company pays no salary, wages, or benefits to the applicant and has no legal liability for any expenses which the applicant incurs as a result of the deceptive orientation they have received.

When searching for employment in the business community, it is always best to begin by utilizing personal contacts. Despite the numerous institutions which exist to assist applicants in their job searches, many new positions are filled as the result of personal contacts between management personnel and people whose opinions they value. Before beginning a job search, the dyslexic graduate should evaluate the resources which are available with respect to personal contacts and attempt to find employment with the assistance of these people. If the dyslexic graduate applies for a job with the recommendation of a person who is known and trusted by management personnel, his chances for employment are greatly enhanced. His chances for employment are greatly diminished if he applies for the position as a stranger who must demonstrate his trustworthiness to the interviewer.

THE DYSLEXIC GRADUATE AND GOVERNMENT EMPLOYMENT

One alternative to corporate employment is government employment. Government positions which are available on the local, state, and federal levels are numerous and require a diversity of college degrees. In addition, the government has a Selective Placement Program to promote the hiring of disabled and minority applicants. Government employment is secure and the benefits are as good or better than those offered within the business community. The only exemptions from the Selective Placement Program are positions within the military and some positions in federal law enforcement agencies. The dyslexic graduate may contact the nearest Office of Personnel Management to obtain current information regarding employment practices which apply to dyslexics.

Government employment offers a dyslexic graduate the opportunity to gain experience which he may use later to obtain employment in the business community. Government employment is a good option for dyslexic graduates because they may benefit from policies which promote the hiring and advancement of applicants who are categorized as being disabled. Whereas the business community might view dyslexia as a hindrance, the government is likely to treat dyslexia as a condition which may be accommodated under governmental employment policy.

If the dyslexic graduate desires a career in the business community which appears unobtainable, a good success strategy is to apply for government employment which offers training in areas related to the desired career. Once the graduate obtains this training and successfully completes two or three years of government employment, he may apply to the business community and obtain the desired position as a result of the training, experience, and possible seniority he has achieved through his government employment.

THE DYSLEXIC ENTREPRENEUR

A third option available to the dyslexic graduate is entrepreneurship. Operating a business can consume a considerable amount of time and money, so careful planning should be done before making a final decision to begin operations. Although the federal government currently has no loan programs directed specifically toward the

72

disabled, the dyslexic entrepreneur should contact the Small Business Administration (SBA) and apply for a Guaranty Loan in which money is borrowed from a commercial lending institution and the SBA assumes responsibility for up to 90% of the loan in the event of default. This procedure reduces the borrower's risk to only 10% of the amount of the loan. The SBA also offers direct loans to entrepreneurs along with business consulting before and after they have begun business. If the dyslexic graduate chooses to become an entrepreneur, he may wish to contact organizations which benefit dyslexics in order to obtain business contacts and promote his products or services.

The dyslexic entrepreneur enjoys the freedom to control his destiny which he would lack as an employee in the business community or government. He is never restricted by policies which conflict with his dyslexia, he is free to work at his own pace, he sets his own schedule, and most importantly, he is free to use his creative abilities without limit. On the other hand, he must finance his business and survive on the revenue it generates. He enjoys no job security and he lives his life as an individual rather than a member of a group.

For the dyslexic graduate, entrepreneurship should be carefully examined if sufficient capital exists to form a business. The dyslexic entrepreneur holds an advantage over his non-dyslexic competitors because he has access to creative abilities which he may use to derive profit and establish himself in the market. Many dyslexics choose to become entrepreneurs after they make several unsuccessful attempts to enter and prosper within traditional institutions. Due to pictorial thought processes, the dyslexic will frequently view the world from a unique perspective and often develop insight from which to benefit as a result of his inability to implement reforms in institutions which are resistant to change. The ability to control ones destiny provides the freedom to act in accordance with ones instincts.

THE DYSLEXIC GRADUATE AND GRADUATE SCHOOL

The fourth option available to the dyslexic graduate is to continue college education in an attempt to receive an advanced degree. This decision should be made only after he has considered how difficult college has been, how he feels about college, and whether or not he is willing to forfeit two years of gainful employment and practical experience to obtain an advanced degree. Graduate students must complete two to three times as much course work as undergraduate students during the same amount of time. If the dyslexic graduate has had difficulty with course work as an undergraduate student, then he probably should not pursue an advanced degree because he may place himself in a situation where he is required to accomplish more than his capabilities will allow. Although he would still have the same rights that he had as an undergraduate, the sheer volume of work could be sufficient to cause him to fail. In addition to extensive course work, many graduate students must serve as teaching assistants for professors in order to graduate. A teaching assistant is responsible for the more mundane tasks involved in teaching a course, such as grading assignments and exams, preparing study sheets, conducting study sessions, and operating office machinery. Being a teaching assistant involves hard work with little praise and considerable responsibility.

If the dyslexic graduate considers graduate school, he must determine whether he would benefit more in two years from the receipt of a masters degree or two years business experience along with the financial compensation which accompanies these efforts. As a graduate student, he could experience financial difficulties because graduate students have little time available for employment and must often rely on scholarships and student loans. As a result, they often graduate in debt and experience pressure to accept employment in unsuitable positions with little or no work experience to offer. If the dyslexic graduate chooses to enter the business community after receiving a bachelors degree, he would have an employment history in two years as well as savings if he is frugal.

I have frequently heard business people say that they prefer an ambitious applicant with a bachelors degree to an average applicant with a masters degree. Some business people even prefer an applicant with a bachelors degree over an applicant with a masters degree. They claim that a person who has spent six years in college is more difficult to train because he has been taught subjects which are based on theory rather than fact. Whether an applicant has a bachelors or a masters degree, he must successfully complete training in order to perform in accordance with business or government expectations and assimilate into the bureaucratic hierarchy.

Regardless of the degree which the dyslexic graduate earns, it may be difficult for him to succeed in his chosen career because he is a unique person who will probably not fit into the organizational mold due to the fact that he thinks differently from most people. After completing a minimum of sixteen years in the American education system, he will probably have experienced conflict with the establishment and be independent and outspoken as a result. Many organizations seek applicants who follow instructions and don't question authority. For this reason, prospective employers may consider dyslexics to be undesirable, regardless of their credentials.

Whatever path the dyslexic student chooses to pursue after graduation, he must realize that he has earned his college diploma and no one can take it away from him. Although the college degree is a key to open doors to the future, the dyslexic graduate must work hard to find a door in which the key will fit. Opportunities are numerous for a creative person who is willing to work hard and take risks. Graduation from college is not an end; it is only the beginning.

EPILOGUE

After having read this book, the reader should realize that the
American education system is neither invincible nor infallible and
that education occurs due to opposition as well as cooperation. Life
is comprised of intricate relationships which must be analyzed and
influenced to satisfy individual needs. The ability to analyze is
developed through study and academic instruction while the ability to
influence, or manipulate, relationships which are present in the
environment is developed as a result of opposition.

Cooperation and opposition compliment each other because they
provide an individual with the ability to function effectively in
order to achieve goals. When an imbalance of the two occurs due to
improper teaching methods or negative self-images, the individual is
unable to function effectively and goals seem unattainable because he
lacks the necessary skills to realize them.

Such has been the case with dyslexics who have been denied proper
academic instruction from modern education systems. Faced with
seemingly insurmountable obstacles, dyslexics have traditionally
responded by using their abilities to manipulate these systems or
fail. In this event, dyslexics who retained positive self-images often
turned to crime in order to achieve goals for which society would
provide no means to realize. Those who suffered the effects of
self-ridicule were permanently disadvantaged due to internal as well
as external limitations.

Education, in its purest form, may be defined as the acquisition
of knowledge which enables an individual to exist in harmony with
others and the environment. It is my sincere desire for the reader to
have found this book to be an educational resource from which to
achieve his goals in life.

HELPFUL ADDRESSES

1) ORTON DYSLEXIA SOCIETY
   Chester Building, Suite 382
   8600 LaSalle Rd.
   Baltimore, MD 21204-6020
   (301) 296-0232

   Contact: Rosemary F. Bowler, Executive Director

2) NATIONAL NETWORK OF LEARNING DISABLED ADULTS
   808 N. 82nd St., Suite F2
   Scottsdale, AZ 85257
   (602) 941-5112

   Contact: Bill Butler

3) LEARNING DISABILITIES ASSOCIATION OF AMERICA
   4156 Library Rd.
   Pittsburgh,PA 15234
   (412) 341-1515

   Contact: Jean Peterson, Executive Director

4) COUNCIL FOR LEARNING DISABILITIES
   P.O. Box 40303
   Overland Park, KS 66204
   (913) 492-8755

   Contact: Kirsten McBride, Executive Secretary

5) NATIONAL CENTER FOR LEARNING DISABILITIES
   99 Park Ave., Sixth Floor
   New York, NY 10016
   (212) 687-7211

   Contact: Arlyn Gardner, Executive Director

6) TIME OUT TO ENJOY
   P.O. Box 1084
   Evanston, IL 60204

INDEX